INNER HEALING

For Deep Wounds Superficially Cured

Gwen A. Washington, D. Min.

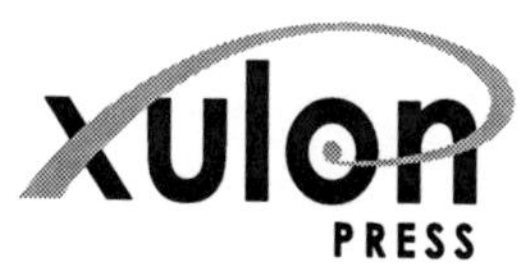

Inner Healing
For Deep Wounds Superficially Cured
by Gwen A. Washington, D. Min.

Printed in the United States of America

ISBN 9781619961814

www.xulonpress.com

CONTENTS

Acknowledgements vii

Introduction
There Is A Set Time for Everything ix

Chapter 1
A Broken Heart Could End In Cardiac Arrest 19

Chapter 2
Identity Crises 45

Chapter 3
Avoid the Grasshopper Mentality: Low Self-Esteem 63

Chapter 4
Be Set Free: Inner Healing 84

Chapter 5
Inner Healing for Wounds Superficially Cured 106

Chapter 6
Wounded Women, Wound Other Women 136

Chapter 7
Signs, Wonders, and Miracles Concerning Healing 171

Notes 195

ACKNOWLEDGEMENTS

With the planting of the first church in the beginning of 1992, I had people who came to my ministry who were wounded from issues in life. Things they may have not been aware of that was stagnating their lives to keep them from reaching their potential. I saw brokenness everyday in our church, at the Wayside Christian Homeless Mission where we ministered for nine years. We saw devastation on the street corners in drug infested communities in Louisville, Kentucky, where residents had allowed gangs, and drug dealers to set up their marketplace right in the neighborhood. They were there to market their dads, moms, sons, daughters, grandfathers, grandmothers, brothers, sisters, uncles, aunts, cousins, the preacher, the worship leader, the choir member, and whoever else they could destroy. We saw so many people with deep wounds who were superficially cured. A great part of my mission as an evangelist, pastor, and teacher was to go the hedges and highways and compel them to come in. This is what we did. I want to thank the Holy Spirit for leading us so many times where to go and what to do when we arrived. I thank God for men and women of God who supported this endeavor, including my husband Elder Arthur Washington, who never tried to block me from doing the mission. I want to thank Faith Christian Life Center Ministries birthed in 1992, and Faith Dominion World Healing Ministries in 2007.

Many were wounded when they came to our ministry but God healed them. Some of those who were birthed from our ministry have become powerful leaders in the Kingdom of God. Thanks a million for my mother, grandmother, and my aunt Norma, especially my grandmother Ethel who taught me the truth and encouraged me about holiness. Thank you Bishop Dennis V. Lyons for the initial ministry preparation, along with the Holy Spirit. It has been a rewarding journey. I am appreciative of Dr. Stephen Rasor, professor of the Doctor of Ministry program at the Interdenominational Theological Center, in Atlanta, who encouraged me in pursuing my passion, to see people healed. To the Full Gospel Baptist Church Fellowship you were a covering for me while I wrote this book, and are my pastors today. Thank you Bishop Paul S. Morton and Dr. Debra Morton, and to others in leadership in FGBCF- Bishop M. L. Priester for a pastor's words of wisdom, Overseer Dr. Marlon Moss for standing with me in whatever move I made, and for Pastor Norman Martin in becoming the pastor for Faith Dominion for me to be released into the "new thing" God has for me. Once again I thank God for my spouse, Arthur who believes in me and supports my endeavors.

I am appreciative of Tarsha Semakula for reading the manuscript initially. I am grateful to Dr. Ada Taylor for editing this manuscript with patience, diligence, preciseness with a spirit of excellence, and for coaching me. Appreciation is extended to the Interdenominational Theological Center professors and to the staff at Xulon Press. A special note of thanks to Robert L. Martin, M.D., for the final editing of my book.

INTRODUCTION

For certain there was another book in me that needed to come out but it was important to wait for the right moment: That moment began one August morning in 2009, as I lay prostrate before the Lord's Presence on my face in the church. *Inner Healing: for Deep Wounds Superficially Cured* was the title given to me, and with it came further instructions concerning a series of books on healing. The Holy Spirit spoke to my spirit, saying: "With the state of healthcare today, your writing will be most sought after; stick to what I reveal to you in secret places." Additional instructions were given that cannot be revealed publicly.

We are in a critical state: the economy, health care, employment, and the emotional-spiritual state of humanity are of grave concern. People need to know that when all of their resources have dried up, there is still hope that exists in this chaotic world. The systems of the world were designed to be temporal, not to last indefinitely. There is another system, one that is perpetual, eternal, absolute, constant, endless, unceasing, and definitely has been established to withstand failing wonders around it—that system represents *the Kingdom of God.*

There are those who have had their day to be popular, highly esteemed, exalted, desired, sought after and emulated.

There are many who have been put on the world's list of the fabulously wealthy, best dressed, most intellectual, biggest donor, or whatever the greatest admirable deed. Affording some such world titles has not decreased the numbers of those living in poverty, has done little to prevent abuse, has yet to stop drug dealers from destroying communities . . . nor convinced pants 'saggers' to "Pull Your Pants Up," as Dooney DaPriest rightfully entreats in his CD.

Band-aids, masks, sunglasses, over-used cosmetics, drugs, alcohol, debasing music, and gang involvements may serve as a cover up but cannot offer a cure for deeply inflicted wounds of the soul. When we allow wounds to heal, but only superficially, we create issues that later become even more problematic. For example, when a person is diagnosed with depression, the first response is to mask it with some type of medication, such as antidepressants. Such pharmaceuticals as these are quick-mood elevators that deal superficially with the issue instead of getting to its root cause—the real problem. Depression is a symptom of deeper inner pain and suffering. Antidepressants are used to mask the signs and symptoms momentarily; however, the real issues have not been dealt with so that complete relief and cure manifest.

Whatever happened to pastoral care and counseling? What happened to the ministry of miracles, deliverances and healings the Father anointed Jesus to operate in? Why are we, the body of Christ, not using the delegated authority Jesus gave to us to bind and loose people from demonic strongholds? Have believers lost compassion for the welfare of others? Why is the Church not doing the greater works that Jesus spoke of in John 14:12: "*Most assuredly, I say to you, he who believes in me, the works that I do he will do also, and greater works than these he will do; because I go to my Father.*"

Did Jesus practice a superficial healing for those He touched . . . or was their problem totally resolved once they came into contact with Him? The time has come for the presence and power of God to manifest throughout the earth, to give people hope in a decaying world. The time has come to uncover the lies told by the adversary to the world. *"Be sober, be vigilant (watchful); because your adversary the devil walks about like a roaring lion, seeking whom he may devour"* (1Peter 5:8 NKJV).

I was exposed to the ministry of healing as a child in the *Church of God in Christ* (COGIC); a Pentecostal church my family attended in the western region of Kentucky. My grandmother and infant cousin were both healed as a result of the Bishop of our organization laying hands on them, and praying for their recovery. They were both healed miraculously—a wonderful experience that will never be forgotten. The experiences from that church have been instrumental in renewing my faith, as it relates to over twenty years of ministry. I have practiced laying hands on the sick and praying for their recovery, whenever the opportunity has arisen. I believe in the supernatural power of God, because I believe first in the God of miracles.

There was an unmistakable healing anointing that covered our church and ministry the first twelve years of my pastorate. In our first church, planted in January 1992, sickness and disease eluded the people who comprised our ministry. We never had a sick or shut-in list; this was truly the hand of God confirming the work He had called us to do for Him. It was the sovereignty of God—not because we had faith enough to conquer anything, but because God upholds everything by the Word of His power. God cannot lie. We believed, and the glory of the Lord manifested in our midst many times. God was molding us to walk by faith, not by sight.

God's favor rested upon the new church. Into its assembly came some possessed and oppressed by demon spirits; it took the power of God to deliver them—and He did! As a new pastor I had to rely on the Holy Spirit to teach me. I knew what the Word of God said, but it took the presence and power of God to put it into action. Fasting, praying, seeking God's face, listening to His voice, and meditating on His Word helped me to begin walking in the ministry of deliverance, healing and restoration. In-depth study of books that taught on deliverance and healing, written by authors who moved in this sacred vein, also afforded me greater wisdom, knowledge, and understanding as to how others operate in these ministry gifts. Of course, the Holy Bible was—and continues to be—my first book of reference, and daily I continue to learn and grow in God's grace. Through the Holy Spirit's leading and guiding, we will reach many souls for Christ with God's message of healing, hope, and restoration—the *good news.*

For approximately twelve years, I served as a pastor before relocating to Atlanta, Georgia in August 2003, taking a three-year sabbatical to complete seminary training at the Interdenominational Theological Center. Before becoming a pastor, I became connected to a ministry that believed in the Holy Spirit and His gifts: signs, wonders and miracles were demonstrated in and through that leader who operated in the gifts of faith, healing, and miracles, among other supernatural powers. My spouse and I personally sowed into that ministry and also sowed from our church finances to cover the people with the same blessings—allowing the healing mantle to rest upon our ministry. The authority and anointing this pastor walked in and practiced consistently flowed from his ministry down to partnering ministries.

Iron does sharpen iron as the Word proclaims: "*Iron sharpens iron; so a man* (woman) *sharpens the countenance of his friend [to show rage or worthy purpose"* (Proverbs 27:17 AMP, insertion mine). It is vitally important to be connected with others who are anointed to operate in the ministry to which you have been called; that the gifts may be stirred up within you. It is necessary to find the stream that our ministry is to flow in and to allow the Spirit to divinely connect us for the supernatural to occur.

The words of this book are being penned in what is now my appointed time to move forward in fulfilling a vision for a world-wide ministry: to preach and teach deliverance to the sick, the diseased and infirmed, as Jesus declared in Luke 4:18,19. God wants to reveal His glory throughout the Universe. He wants to use His people, whom He has anointed, to do great feats. It is our appointed time to witness to how God does miracles through the presence and the power of the Holy Spirit abiding in men and women, girls and boys. *"Jesus said to him, "If you can believe, all things are possible to him* (her) *who believes*" (Mark 9:23 NKJV, insertion mine).

Faith Healing Ministry: A Christian Education Model for Clergy and Laity was the focus of my dissertation; a study and search into why during the 21st Century there is a lack of faith healing in the Christian church. Most mainline Christian churches do not have healing as a recognized ministry—mainly due to a mistaken belief that miracles ceased after the first century. Sixteenth century reformers taught that the Word of God has precedence (rank) over the gifts of God. Now it is up to those who believe, and will obey the call today, to go forth and demonstrate that the Holy Spirit is present in us to act in Christ's behalf. He empowers us for a season and a reason to bless others.

The body of Christ has been given different gifts; not everyone has the same gifts. Apostle Paul charged believers, "*But earnestly desire the best gifts, and yet I show you a more excellent way*" (1 Corinthians 12:31). The gifts of the Holy Spirit will remain on the earth as God wills; therefore, we must use them to equip, edify and bless God's people. There are individuals, who have not yet come into the knowledge of the truth about the Lord Jesus being Savior and Redeemer, who will believe in Him through experiencing signs, wonders and miracles.

> *So He came to Nazareth, where He had been brought up. And as His custom was, He went into the synagogue on the Sabbath day, and stood up to read. And He was handed the book of the prophet Isaiah. And when He had opened the book, He found the place where it was written: The Spirit of the LORD is upon Me, because He has anointed me to preach the gospel to the poor; He has sent Me to heal the broken hearted, to proclaim liberty to the captives and recovery of sight to the blind, to set at liberty those who are oppressed; To proclaim the acceptable year of the LORD (Luke 4:16-19 NKJV).*

Isaiah, as well as other prophets, was looking for the deliverance and restoration of God's people from Babylonian captivity. The expected deliverance would release slaves, restore property rights, and cancel all debts. Moreover, the reference pertained to the future *Messianic Age*, the coming of Jesus the Son of God, and of His kingdom.

All debts were cancelled when Jesus took on the sins of the world to liberate humanity. The stripes Jesus received represent our healing through His suffering and crucifixion! According to *Strong's Concordance*, the Greek word *kairos* means "for an occasion, set or proper time, season, opportunity, or due time." It was Jesus' set time to come forth in Luke 4:18, 19; it had been prophesied seven hundred years before by the prophet Isaiah. When destiny calls, it propels you to go forth because favor has preceded you. Now is our destined time—our *kairos* moment.

This book, *Inner Healing for Deep Wounds Superficially Cured*, compares a person who is broken on the inside to one who is in cardiac arrest; the potential for death to occur can happen in both cases. Without help in bringing about a healing, inner wounds can lead to a person committing spiritual or natural suicide, or wounding others. Cardiac arrest can lead to death due to cessation of breathing and all heart functions.

Some individuals have issues with their identity, resulting from deep wounds which may stem from abuse, neglect, or other forms of misuse. Discussion is given to how the Israelites were unable to come into their promise due to their need for inner healing. They could not see themselves liberated because of the slave mentality they had been accustomed to for generations, which amounted to approximately four hundred and thirty years. They were wounded on the inside, spiritually and emotionally—in memories, thoughts, and feelings. These issues were further impacted by physical toil and forced labor, depleting the Israelites of their strength. They needed deliverance from rejection, anger, disappointment, strife, unforgiveness, bitterness and other inner hurts.

Their wounds could have been healed through trusting God and their spiritual leader, who walked in close communion with God. God had means for them to receive their cure, as He has provided the same for us today. God intervenes supernaturally; we can receive divine intervention through healing prayers, biblical counseling, and by developing a personal relationship with Him while waiting in expectancy. The Israelites suffered from lack of confidence in God, in their leader, and in themselves. Due to past experiences of pain and suffering, they did not learn to completely trust others. It is important to discuss the Israelites because they had the potential to excel but failed because of their defeated mental image of God and self. Out of all those who were brought out of Egypt, only two, Joshua and Caleb were able to reach the Promise Land.

Via my pastoral experiences, I reflect here on how wounded people—superficially cured—can cause havoc inside as well as outside the church. People who are always suffering from inner hurt are those who cannot let go of the past. Discussion is also given herein to some family issues—personal experiences with rejection, anger, unforgiveness and other painful situations. It had been my experience to hurt or wound others because of having been wounded myself. I had to learn to release anger, resentment, feelings of rejection, bitterness, strife, and unforgiveness in order to move forward. Inner healing involves letting go of past thoughts, feelings, affections, desires, intentions, memories, and other situations in order to be set free. For me, it was a process; it did not happen overnight.

Many seemingly wish for instant results all the time to avoid the stages of healing; however, it is necessary that we allow deep wounds to go through the full process of healing and recovery. This is not to suggest that healing cannot be instantaneous, for God does heal miraculously! As one goes through various stages of healing, you are able to learn patience and develop a trusting relationship with God, and with your mentor. Developing trusting relationships is of upmost importance during the healing process; you need someone to coach you through to completion. As you experience stages of healing, you will also encounter a loving, gentle, kind, good and faithful God who never leaves you without hope: "*Being confident of this very thing, that He who has begun a good work in you will complete it until the day of Jesus Christ*" (Philippians1:6 NKJV). To have a totally successful recovery, wounds must be healed from the internal to external.

1

A BROKEN HEART *and* POSSIBLE CARDIAC ARREST

A cardiac (heart) arrest means that your heart has stopped functioning or a cessation of cardiac capacity has occurred. When this happens in a medical facility, you have qualified men and women who answer to the code call immediately—often times a 'Code Blue' or 'Code 100.' Trained medical staff knows that within 3 to 6 minutes of a cardiac arrest, the victim may suffer irreversible brain damage; therefore, the crash cart, defibrillator, ambu bag, ventilator, and other emergency equipment are brought to the room STAT—immediately, without delay. Medical as well as non-medical staffers, such as physicians, nurses, respiratory therapists, lab technicians, and others who have been trained to respond to life-threatening situations react swiftly to save a life.

Some methods successfully employed to save life are cardioversion, ventilation, cardiopulmonary resuscitation (CPR), and insertion of intravenous lines to instill emergency medications. Is it not just as important to save someone who is broken in spirit? Without the proper support, a brokenhearted person could very easily end up as a cardiac-arrest victim.

Irregular rhythms of the ventricles can lead to cardiac arrest. We see people every day who experience cardiac dysfunction: the physical heart is not functioning normally and from an EKG or electrocardiogram, the rhythm is determined to be irregular. Whether it is one's physical heart or the inner heart of a person, it needs to have normal function without compromise to get the best output. The ventricles contract so that blood can be pumped from the physical heart throughout the body. When the ventricles are diseased, they may suffer *tachycardia* (fast heartbeat), flutter (the heart is flapping but ineffective), or go into ventricular fibrillation (rapid, irregular, chaotic rhythm), or into fatal cardiac standstill. There is always a process before reaching the point where no cardiac activity exists.

So many are those who are suffering from inner pain and shame! Just as a physical heart that is poorly functioning requires immediate attention, so does a person who has suffered from a broken heart. Remember, a physical heart that is diseased or sustains damage from a *Myocardial Infarction* (heart attack), or other insults, will not survive unless the matter is attended to immediately. Many times no emergency team is available to help in discerning the needs of those suffering, nor is there immediate aid in times of distress. Some find temporary relief by abusing prescription medications, or may overdose on street drugs looking for relief; others try escapism through various forms of suicide.

Still there are some who literally give up trying and resort to crime, street life, or deep depression, with an inability to function in a normal, everyday mode. Many resort to living on the streets (a homeless lifestyle), because they cannot cope with life's challenges alone. These types of individuals are usually rejected, pushed away by relatives because their coping mechanisms may be unacceptable to the bureaucrats of the family. It is a sad indictment against the family to have loved ones who feel so rejected or so out of place that they will separate from their family of origin—live among strangers in the streets, or in some homeless shelter. Except for the grace of God, it could be you or I!

Many times, the biological family is the first to renounce a loved one who is different or demonstrates unacceptable behavior. Certainly, there are some relatives who pose unrealistic challenges that are difficult to cope with, but there are others who just need a helping hand to get out of a slump. We all have those kinds of relatives that we want to forget, that we may be ashamed of, but remember that rejection is difficult to overcome; some never heal from the wounds of repeated renunciation.

It is so sad how emotions you dealt with as a child will try to provoke you even in your adult life. I have experienced rejection so many times in my childhood as well as in adulthood. Many times it is because one has not dealt with issues experienced as a child or adolescent; they are masked or temporarily covered with masking tape. Covering them up then becomes problematic! It is usually the pain, shame and hurt that you do not want to face, but it is important to allow it to surface to receive your deliverance and inner healing.

Repeated disappointments can alter one's sense of security about themselves and others. Oftentimes as a child you are made to feel as if you have done something wrong, and that is why others do not follow through with promises to you. At times you may find yourself reverting to defense mechanisms or barriers used as a child to protect your inner self. These things may have helped then; however, it is now time to come out of the shell and face the issues head on. Many commit suicide or plan to take their life or even that of another because of perceived failure, rejection, disappointment, and an inability to cope with unexpected changes in life.

We are living in a time where the giants of this world are leaving here fast; things that we once thought were stable are crumbling all around us. The economic status of our nation is in a disheartened place, but God has promised to never leave us nor forsake us. These distressing times did not take Him by surprise. We are warned in the Bible that distressing times will come.

If we study and meditate on the Word of God, we will find that biblical prophecy is being fulfilled right before our eyes. Things in this world will not improve, but you can improve as a believer in Christ because He promised: *"A thousand may fall at your side, and ten thousand at your right hand side, but it shall not come near you"* (Psalm 91:7 NKJV).

As a child I suffered internally because of being a person who did not want anyone to know how she felt, or the things I desired to see changed in my life. Cutting pictures of men, women, and children out of catalogues and displaying them with paper furniture helped to portray what I envisioned as the ideal family and home life. I did not openly discuss my desires but rather held onto those images of my heart and mind. My 'paper doll' images continued well into my teen years.

I felt rejected as a child because my parents were separated; they both lived out of our home in a city two hundred miles away. It was difficult for me to understand why my friends lived in a home with their parents, while my siblings and I lived separate from our parents. My paternal grandmother raised her son's children without support from him; we had to survive off of two hundred, thirty-five dollars a month, because there was no 'food stamp' support during my childhood. There was governmental dispensed sharp cheese, along with powdered milk, powdered eggs, yellow corn meal, pulled pork in a can, and possibly another item just as tasteless. Yet my grandmother and aunt always managed to feed us well!—government food was not our usual way of eating. Grandmother would charge food items every month and pay for them when the check arrived.

My grandmother and aunt did not mistreat us; they gave us love and cared for our well-being. Still I cried almost every night for my family to be together; I just wanted to be in a home with both parents present, because the majority of my school friends lived with both parents. Little did I understand then that being in my grandmother's home was the best situation for us, my siblings and me.

Dad was an alcoholic who was abusive to my mother. I remember once when my dad and mother just happened to be in my grandmother's home at the same time (both were living in Louisville, but not together in the same house). I was sleeping in between them and was suddenly awakened by my mother responding to my dad's selfish request. He began striking my mother with his hands, and when I cried out Grandmother intervened to stop his abusive behavior. I was so hurt and disappointed in him. It was an answer to my cry for my parents to be together, but my dad blew it!—again, I felt rejected!

I remember as a child having to wear my grandmother's shoes to school because my only pair was worn completely out. Hers were too narrow for my feet so I busted out the back of them and had to use a piece of wire to hold the seams together. The soles wore out while I waited to receive new shoes from my father. In the meantime I had to cut a lining for my shoes from a box in order to keep my feet from touching the ground. Eventually, my dad sent to me a pair of black shoes and two pairs of socks, one blue and the other rose colored. Until I became grown, that is all I remember receiving from my dad as a child.

My skin color was not like that of my dad, brother or younger sister. Dad passed for a Caucasian when African-Americans, or colored people (as we were called back then), could not ride in the front of the bus or drink from the same water fountain as whites. He was able to get employment where most blacks were denied work because of their skin color. Most of Dad's family was 'light-skinned'—of mixed Indian and Caucasian ancestry. I felt different growing up because of my skin color; mine came from my mother's side of the family which averaged from brown to 'dark-skinned.' At those times that I especially felt different, my feelings were suppressed; I did not learn to share or discuss them with others. By holding in these feelings I developed thoughts of inferiority about matters in my life, always feeling ashamed during my growing up years.

My brother Bob was never ashamed to tell people that we were underprivileged. Eventually he moved away . . . went on to complete medical school . . . now lives in Hawaii with his spouse, Christina, where he serves as a physician. Bob has done well in his profession. He comes back to Kentucky two to three times a year to be with the family. There was a time I would be so embarrassed when Bob would invariably speak these words: "We were so poor coming up." I wanted to jump up and put my hand over his mouth! I had not dealt with the issue of being underprivileged during our growing-up years; it was a part of my past I wanted to forget.

If you do not allow issues to surface so they can be dealt with properly, you may find yourself walking in shame or overcompensating in a particular area. I became a spendthrift in the areas of moving from one home to another and in spending money I did not have. And even as an adult, I stilled walked in denial! Even today, I enjoy giving to help others—especially to advance the kingdom of God; sometimes, my husband believes I go overboard in giving.

As stated previously, I did not want to feel even more ashamed by allowing others to know my thoughts, how I felt on the inside. This resulted in inner suffering which manifested in nail biting, bed wetting, crying at night, feeling rejection, withdrawal, shame, and anger—all symptomatic of being wounded as a child. Some people may not believe that parents separating and getting divorced has a devastating impact on their children, but it does! I understand in some cases that separation or divorce may prove necessary because of domestic violence, or such; however, if it can be avoided, for the sake of the children, it is worth trying to work matters out.

Besides being a bed wetter, an issue where I experienced shame, I was also faced with being overweight for my age—creating yet another issue: my weight was approximately180 pounds as a young teen. Our family ate good meals, and maybe that was my grandmother's way of compensating for our lack in other things. We were able to eat well, because Grandmother was able to charge groceries until the government-issued check arrived each month. My aunt worked at Fort Campbell, Kentucky laundering clothes for the soldiers, and with her income we survived.

Because I was extremely quiet, children often teased me, and some had a tendency to say outright negative things about me. I felt rejected but tried to hide the hurt . . . and, although I was not a bully, I resorted to fighting when I figured I had taken too much. There were some youths around my age who were known bullies, wanting to tease and fight just for the sake of proving something to themselves. Maybe they were insecure in certain areas . . . we all were in different stages of growth and development.

My grandmother kept us in church, which surely was one of the best things that could have ever happened to my siblings and me. One half of my family was Pentecostal and the other Baptist; nevertheless, we were faithful in attendance and my siblings and I enjoyed working in the church. My involvement in church helped me to overcome some of my obstacles; it was there I learned at an early age to pray to God . . . to trust in Him to come through for me. I had to believe that God would hear and answer my prayers, especially when our clothes and toys from my mother did not arrive until Christmas Eve. We lived on the edge many times, but the Lord was faithful! The Word of God says, "*Train up a child in the way he should go, and when he is old he will not depart from it*" (Proverbs 22:6). My earlier training was instrumental in helping me to turn back to God as a young adult.

Even with my grandmother teaching us how to conduct ourselves as people of integrity, there was something missing in my life; that missing 'something' seduced me to look for love in all the wrong places. It is good to talk to someone about your internal issues, but I was not one to discuss my inner thoughts and feelings. Remember, I was ashamed for anyone to know how I felt on the inside. Let me encourage you to be open, always find someone you trust and talk to them for the release of that inner turmoil. I suppose one of the reasons I hid my feelings and thoughts was because my grandmother and aunt were good to us; therefore, I did not want to seem ungrateful.

In contrast to my feeling ashamed to discuss my inner feelings with anyone, brother Bob seemed to cope well, exhibiting no outwardly manifested symptoms of inner suffering and pain. Our younger brother Stewart was somewhat quiet but became very angry whenever we teased him—to the point of trying to forcibly strike us. Rage came out of him only when he was extremely upset; as children we saw the rage and provoked him even further. Stewart had issues of anger into his early adult life which he overcame. Today, he is a totally different person and currently serves as a deacon in the church my son Norman pastors.

My sister Carolyn was taken to Louisville to live with our mother. I missed her terribly after she moved away; once again it felt that someone close to me had been snatched away—leaving me with further hurt and pain. My siblings and I spent time with our mother during the summer months, and usually at Christmas, or whenever she could get some time off from her employer to visit us. My dad by now was out of the picture. He lived his life as if he did not have a care in the world; he forgot that his mother and sister had put their lives on hold to take care of his responsibilities. I mention the above siblings because these were my dad's children reared by his mother and sister.

Betty, my eldest sister, lived in Louisville with my mother and her family. My maternal grandmother and aunts assisted Mother with Betty's care. Later on my mother had two more children and also remarried. Our stepdad assisted my mother in financially supporting her children; he was more supportive than our biological father.

What was missing in my life was a father to love and counsel me, to be a role model—what a man, husband, and father should be in the life of a girl growing up. Every female child needs her dad as much as does a male child; they both need positive role models. There are some things a father can teach a female child that can help her to overcome pitfalls of life. To know the love of a caring father during childhood helps children not to feel as if there is a void in their lives. My grandmother tried to shelter me, but I became very rebellious and stubborn by age sixteen. I suffered from being heartbroken . . . covered it with a 'band aid,' so that no one would know how I truly felt.

The first time a man told me he loved me it sounded good, because I had never had a man to tell me that before. Satan has all kinds of traps for young folk who are hurting on the inside. No one could help me because I refused to trust and let anyone in my space. I kept a mask on to cover up my pain. If you want to be delivered, take the mask off . . . become transparent! It is important for you to not be ashamed of your inner struggles; someone else has been through what you are experiencing.

I went through years of suffering from an identity crisis, because I failed to heed the training received from my grandmother and rebelled by doing the opposite of what she taught. I befriended certain girls whose parents did not seem to mind if they dated or went to parties, or even stayed out late at night. They were high-school students, who were already engaged in a destructive lifestyle; it was not long before I started hanging out with them, engaging in the same activity as they were engaged in-sneaking around and lying to my grandmother. Even though I was repeatedly reprimanded, it became my habit to come home late into the night.

This "church girl" became so disobedient that I caused my grandmother and aunt a lot of pain and shame. I drank alcohol, went to nightclubs, used profanity, dated an older man and had sex with him. Eventually I had two children by this man, who was twelve years older than I. I thought my grandmother was old fashioned and did not want me to have any fun; little did I realize how much she was concerned about my welfare, and rightfully so. Calling me by my nick-name, she often spoke this reminder: "Titto, you have a good name; you don't need to run with those girls. Their mothers do not care what they do." Grandmother was right!

Reflecting over my life, I now realize that everything my grandmother and aunt taught me was for my own good. It is my regret that I did not heed Grandmother's teachings and use her as my role model, yet in spite of pitfalls, I believe that God never took his hands off of me. God allowed my grandmother to always have open arms of love extended to me even when I acted contrary to her expectations. She and my aunt loved my children and assisted me with their care but insisted that I was not to be with their father. We were not married and he was one who would not have been faithful in marriage at that time. Although eventually he married and became a 'good husband' to his wife, he has never supported the children he fathered with me—who occasionally visit him in Cadiz, Kentucky. I forgave him a long time ago and am grateful that we were not married—convinced my purpose would have been aborted.

God blessed me with good, male role models and support for my children, particularly their uncles and my husband. My children and I were very blessed to have them as role models. It was not to the degree that the children needed, but still they had support of loving men in their lives during their childhood and adolescence. Just as I had done in my youth, my youngest son, Shawn, rebelled . . . possibly because he was not around his dad either. After we divorced (necessary because of his heavy alcohol use and history of physical abuse), his dad no longer supported him. They saw each other only on rare occasions, and when Shawn was sixteen years old, his dad died from cancer. I visited him with Shawn after his initial surgery and also felt the leading of the Holy Spirit to visit him again one Wednesday evening following our Bible class. We interceded for John, and he was born again in Christ! I could not be bitter toward him for not assuming his role as a true husband and a father to his child; instead, I forgave him. When I went to his mother's home to visit with him, it was as if domestic violence had not even been a thorn in our marriage. This is the way we are to be toward those who have hurt us: We must ask Christ to help us to forgive.

God had a plan for my life. Satan, the enemy of my soul wanted to destroy me because he knew one day I would turn back to the Lord. The Holy Spirit reminds me of my grandmother who was always willing_to forgive me for my poor judgment and selfishness. No matter what sins you have committed, Jesus paid the price for them—and I am a living witness. Many times people try to put sin in a category, such as 'big sins' or 'little sins'; there is no such thing—sin is sin, no matter how you spell it! What is important is that Jesus took upon Himself all the sins of humankind and carried them to the cross. Confess your sins to Him and be delivered and healed in whatever area you are hurting!

> *Confess your trespasses (faults) to one another, and pray one for another that you may be healed. The*

effective, fervent prayer of a righteous man avails much" (James 5:16 NKJV). Confess your sins to each other and pray for each other so God can heal you, when a believing person prays, great things happen (James 5:16 NCV).

Confess your sins to each other and pray for each other so that you can Live together whole and healed. The prayer of a person living right with God is something to be reckoned with. Elijah, for instance, human just like us, prayed hard that it would not rain and it did not—not a drop for three and a semi years (James 5:16, 17 The Message Bible).

Jesus said He came to heal the brokenhearted, which indicated the seriousness of the problem, just one of the concerns Jesus addressed when He began His earthly ministry. He knew that a broken person was an incapacitated person, incapable of living an effective life. "*The spirit of a man* (woman) *will sustain his* (her) *infirmity; but a wounded spirit who can bear?*" (Proverbs 18:14, insertion mine). The Word of God emphasizes God's concern for those who have a broken heart: "*The Lord is near to those who have a broken heart, and saves such as have a contrite spirit*" (Psalm 34:18 NKJV).

Why is the Lord near to those who have a broken heart? Remember, those broken in heart represent the character of the righteous in God—persons who are self-emptied and low in their own eyes, having no confidence in their own ability. Their confidence is in the Almighty God, the Creator of the Universe. They are a representation of Jesus, who humbled Himself to leave heaven for earth; to be born of a woman of low status; to suffer the most painful, degrading, humiliating death on a cross by the hands of cruel Roman soldiers. The brokenhearted, addressed in this book, refers to those who may be broken or wounded from losses, repeated insults, continual rejection, broken promises, and physical, emotional or sexual abuse.

The spirit is the life of a person. *Strong's* Concordance asserts that the human spirit is sometimes characterized as the seat of emotions, the mind, and the will. The Greek word for the human heart is *kardia,* the chief organ of the physical life, occupying the most important place in the human system. The inner being of a person—their heart—includes their motives, feelings, affections, desires, and also their will, principles, aims, thoughts and intellect. Regarding the heart then as the seat of emotions, we recognize that there are merry hearts, fearful hearts and troubled hearts. Memory is also regarded as the activity of the heart.

Since the spirit of a person represents the life of an individual, if that spirit or heart is broken, it needs immediate attention. In Luke 4:18 the Word declares that Jesus came to heal the brokenhearted. Here "brokenhearted" means to be completely crushed; to be shattered, bruised, broken in pieces, in shivers, or to break. A broken-hearted person is one who has little hope or who cannot seem to rise above their situation. A quick blow or repeated insults can cause one to become brokenhearted.

The Book of Ruth in the Hebrew Bible (or Old Testament) is very significant because it is a beautiful story of love, loyalty and redemption. It reveals how Ruth transitioned from one culture to another, from serving many gods to serving one God, and her loyalty to a woman who had lost hope. It also reveals how faithfulness to God, loyalty to a person, and obedience, will open doors of favor that can change the entire course of one's purpose for living.

I believe Naomi and her daughter-in-law Ruth suffered from being brokenhearted due to their heavy losses: Naomi had previously left Bethlehem with a husband and two sons to live in Moab, a foreign land; the family left their native country due to a famine in the earth. While dwelling in Moab, the two sons Mahlon and Kilion both married Moabite women. Tragedy occurred in Naomi's household when her husband, Elimelech, died as well as her two sons. I enjoy reading the book of Ruth; it reveals not only their sufferings but how they were able to cope, and also how God intervened in their lives to bring restoration. Jesus is not mentioned in the account of Ruth, but it was chosen as one of the sixty-six canonical books of the Bible. Boaz (who becomes husband to Ruth) is a type of Christ; he was both Ruth and Naomi's redeemer, just as Christ is our Savior and Redeemer.

The Jews, God's chosen people, rejected Him, which gave us, the Gentiles, an opportunity to receive salvation. Naomi, a Jew, was one of God's chosen people. Ruth, a Gentile, heard about this God that Naomi worshiped and constantly talked about, then believed and received Him as her God. Ruth demonstrated her faith in the God of Naomi by leaving behind Moab and the Moabite gods.

The *Targum*, a Jewish translation of the Hebrew Bible, informs us that Naomi's sons died from transgressing (breaking) the law in marrying foreign women. This is likely if they went into idolatry with the Moabites. One thing is clear from the Hebrew Law: long life was promised if the law was obeyed, and the cutting off of life if it was disobeyed. In Deuteronomy 7:2, 3, God instructed the Israelites (the Hebrews) to smite the nations and utterly destroy them, make no covenant with them, show them no mercy, and make no marriage with them. Do not give your daughters to them (Dake's Bible).

While writing this book, I viewed a televised film on Trinity Broadcasting Network (TBN) about the story of Ruth. This adaptation of Ruth's story portrayed her younger son Mahlon's attraction to Ruth and desire to be with her, depicting how he was forbidden to enter the king's palace to see Ruth. She, at the time, was going through her purification rites in order to come before the king. As the movie continued, Mahlon's desire to see Ruth was made known to the Moabite king, who then sent soldiers to the family's home and took into custody Elimelech and his elder son Kilion. Both men were killed. Mahlon was severely injured later in his attempt to take Ruth out of the king's court; although he succeeded and was able to marry Ruth, he died shortly afterwards.

Can you imagine the brokenness Naomi experienced upon losing her spouse and two sons? According to Jewish custom, if a man died and left his wife, and they had a male child, that son was to support his mother. This woman lost both sons—her only means of financial support, therefore losing everything. Their deaths were very heart breaking and devastating for both Naomi and Ruth. When Naomi heard that God had blessed His people by coming to their aid with food, she prepared to return home to Bethlehem. Naomi was not leaving Moab the way she came in; she was leaving alone, except with a stranger of another culture who had married her son. But now they both were widows—broken women, women in need of comfort, financial support, encouragement and acceptance.

Ruth left her home, culture, and religion to come to a new land of foreign people with different beliefs and values—to serve their Hebrew God. It took fortitude, strength, faith, and determination in order for Ruth to enter into another culture that did not accept the Moabites as covenant partners.

I am sure Ruth knew that, somehow, Naomi and she were divinely connected to each other's destiny. Ruth did not have the master plan but she recognized that she was in covenant (agreement, compact, league), through marriage with Naomi's son Mahlon before his death. This made her covenant with Naomi and Naomi's God one Ruth did not wish to break. It reminds me of the God we serve: He is a covenant keeper—God will not break his covenant with us! Naomi had lost her entire family; therefore, she was heartbroken. All Ruth had when she entered Bethlehem was love, respect, and loyalty for her mother-in-law and for the God Naomi worshiped and served. Continuity of these attributes is enough to give one hope when the situation looks hopeless.

By the time she reached Judea, Naomi had little confidence that her circumstances would improve. When the women there greeted her, she could only reply, *"Don't call me Naomi . . . Call me Mara, because the Almighty has made my life very bitter. I went away full, but the LORD has brought me back empty. Why call me Naomi? The LORD has afflicted me; the Almighty has brought misfortune upon me*" (Ruth 1:20, 21 NIV). It appears that Naomi was blaming God for her misfortune; this often happens when tragedy or misfortune occurs. As my grandmother has repeated many times in the past, "There are two sides to every story."

Going back to the thrust of the movie: Who was responsible for aggravating the Moabite king? Israel was in moral decay, apostasy, and oppression at the time of the famine, when Elimelech moved his family there. There was hostility between the Israelites and the Moabites. It was probably not wise for Elimelech to take his family to Moab, but the grass looked greener on the other side. Within ten years of living in Moab, the men of Naomi's family were deceased.

Naomi's heart ceased to function in forgiveness, love, and gentleness; rather she became bitter. Not at all gentle with the women who greeted her upon her return—calling her Naomi, she sternly announced that they were not to call her by her birth name but "Mara," meaning "*bitter.*" It is "appropriate for one whose life was grievous and bitter" (Dake's Bible).

Perhaps Naomi's bitterness rested in a failure to forgive her spouse for taking the family to Moab. Perhaps Naomi blamed God for her perceived notion that He was partly responsible for the death of her family. She may have blamed God for allowing the famine to occur . . . the Moabites for their cruelty to her family. She was returning home as a broken woman with little hope of restoration. Naomi was at the time experiencing inner brokenness, shame, pain, and possibly she felt rejected by the God in whom she trusted. Little did Naomi remember that God always has a 'ram in the bush'—He is a God of healing . . . a God of hope . . . a God of restoration.

In the case of Naomi and Ruth, time was important; any hastiness would not help the women recover the hurt of their losses. Yet time in the story of Ruth is not of the essence as it is during a cardiac arrest, for during a cardiac arrest, speed in responding is critical for the recovery of the patient. Yes, time was very important for Naomi's recovery, but it could not be rushed. She needed time for her broken heart to heal; thus, it was necessary for her to release her bitterness and unforgiveness.

For some people, the time required for healing and recovery may be longer than for others. It is not that God cannot deliver and heal supernaturally; this may depend on how willing a person is to let go of the hurt and pain they are experiencing to be set free. Healing needs to occur from the inside out to prevent wounds from being superficially cured. We do not want wounds covered with a 'band-aid' and that are so infected inwardly, hemorrhaging occurs with the least amount of pressure.

Naomi was able to ventilate—to talk about how she felt on the inside; she let her old friends know that she was bitter . . . did not conceal what she was experiencing and even confessed her faults to them. Her openness gave her friends an opportunity to know what to ask for as they prayed secretly to God to heal Naomi's broken heart. Ruth must have been just as heart-broken as her mother-in-law, but she knew that in order for them to survive, someone had to be responsible for their livelihood.

The story of Ruth and Naomi is a prime example of how God will provide for those who are brokenhearted. Remember, Jesus came to preach, to teach, and to heal the brokenhearted. Jesus is concerned about those who hurt, and especially those wounded internally. Some wounds are covered superficially for a short period; however long, whatever is happening on the inside will eventually be made known on the outside. Sometimes it may be demonstrated in such outward signs as: anger, bitterness, sadness, withdrawal, rebellion, stubbornness, feelings of rejection, low self esteem, low self worth, addictions to sex, food, drugs, alcohol, and cigarettes, control, suicidal tendencies, obsessive, aggressive or compulsive behavior, and relationship issues.

Hold on, help is on the way! If you want to be delivered, call on the name of the Lord. Tell Him you are tired of living as you have been and that you desire to be released. This is the promise stated in the Word of God:

> *The Word is near you, in your mouth and in your heart. That if you confess with your mouth the Lord Jesus and believe in your heart that God has raised Him from the dead, you will be saved. For with the heart one believes unto righteousness, and with the mouth confession is made unto salvation. Whoever calls on the name of the Lord shall be saved* (Romans 10:8b-10, 13 NKJV).

Sometimes after an individual has suffered a heart attack, surgery may be necessary to correct those blocked arteries because they hinder the flow of blood. Once the blockage is removed, the heart can again function as it was created to do; oxygenated blood can flow through the lungs, heart, and throughout the body. Coronary arteries are now free of debris—stuff and junk that may cause blood circulation to cease.

Likewise, the inner heart of an individual must be free of debris for that person to be whole. We concentrate on the body but many times the inner person is a messed up 'piece of junk.' It is time now to teach and practice holistic salvation: spirit, soul, and body. Neglecting the inner person in the deliverance process may become an issue later on or problematic for any individual attempting to fulfill purpose.

Find a mentor who will assist you in keeping your channels clean and open, for destiny is calling. Too many people have aborted their vision, dream, or purpose by failing to guard their heart with all diligence; so find a strong, prayer partner to assist in your deliverance and pursuit. You are spirit . . . live in a body . . . and have a soul. Keep your heart pure; have a daily house cleansing: confess, repent, get purged, and allow the Holy Spirit to refill and refresh you. "*Repent therefore and be converted, that your sins may be blotted out, so that times of refreshing may come from the presence of the Lord, and that He may send Jesus Christ, who was preached to you before*" (Acts 3:19, 20 NKJV).

You are not defeated—as a matter of fact you are coming out a winner! Once you begin to digest the Word of God and get revelation from the Holy Spirit, you will see yourself liberated. You have overcome by the blood of the Lamb and by the word of your testimony. You are victorious, more than a conqueror! You are the head and not the tail. You are above, only, and not beneath. Study and think deeply upon God's blessings of obedience given through Moses to the Israelites in Deuteronomy 28:1-14.

The Book of Ruth is a journey of suffering which contains a joyous ending. In it Naomi does not try to hide her frustrations and pain but, rather, exhibits genuineness and transparency, as do some. Having a whole life makes confessing your faults to one another necessary so that you may be healed; falsifying one's condition only delays the deliverance-healing process. You too have gone through some pits of life, but the Lord has not failed you. God has sustained you, so that you may tell your testimony to another brother or sister—one deceived into believing they are alone in their suffering. Today is your day for a miracle; God has a blessing with your name on it!

You are not alone, and God is with you as much as you will allow Him to be. He is a very present help in the time of trouble. If a broken, angry, bitter, poverty-stricken Hebrew woman and a foreign, despised, Moabite woman could find their way to a land of promise, provision and prosperity, then surely the Lord will do no less for you. Ruth refused to sit in a pity-party group waiting for someone to put something in her hands; she went to work. She was industrious, hard working, and expecting a blessing. God had already established a way for her and Naomi to survive; Ruth had to take the initiative to work the plan God had for her. In the land of promise lies your destiny and you will obtain the stamina, through prayer, to rise up and declare victory rather than defeat. Pray in the Spirit . . . and with the Spirit rise above your situation . . . then follow the plan God lays out for you.

The Lord has come to heal your broken heart. He did it for Naomi and Ruth and He will do it for you. Who told you to sink down into despair? It is time for the true soldiers of the Lord to stand up. You will, at times, become battle fatigued, but your Help is always present. God, the Almighty will send help from the sanctuary and strengthen you out of Zion, His Holy Hill (or His dwelling in heaven): "*May the LORD answer you in the day of trouble; May the name of the God of Jacob defend you; May He send you help from the sanctuary, And strengthen you out of Zion*" (Psalm 20:1, 2 NKJV). When you are facing circumstances that try to overwhelm you cry out to the Lord, He will hear you and answer in your times of distress. He will send someone to assist you during your time of need; it may be through encouraging words or a prayer of faith.

Confess the Word of God over your life; God honors His Word. Anything broken can be repaired or put back together again. You may have to go to the "potter's house" for Him to break you all over again and to remold you according to His divine plan. He will do it just for you. You have a choice in determining your path to restoration and wholeness.

Satanic forces will try to make your situation seem hopeless; do not allow your brokenness to oppress you. People often suffer losses from death, unemployment, separation, divorce, and bad relationships; such losses do not have to bring stagnation in pursuit of one's harvest, one's dreams. Allow your brokenness to be a place of preparation for the next dimension of God's divine will to be made known. God always has a greater plan . . . He does know the end from the beginning. Praise God, through to your victory!

Remember, Ruth and Naomi had to leave a place of brokenness to discover their place of promise, provision, and prosperity. God had prepared a Boaz for Ruth . . . and Naomi would ultimately benefit from it, proving that God rewards the faithful. Ruth forsook all to follow the God who created the heavens and earth, the only true and living God of all life. She demonstrated high moral character in her kindness, loyalty, and faithfulness to Naomi, and to Naomi's God. Her place of pain became her place of gain; her misery—her ministry. She could unashamedly, unapologetically say, "Look, what the Lord has done! He is my Kinsman Redeemer, my perpetual Father and Eternal Savior."

Women, be encouraged and wait on your Boaz; get yourself in position, that God may favor you. Ruth positioned herself and met Boaz by gleaning (picking up) grain in his field.

> *And Ruth the Moabitess said unto Naomi, Let me now go to the field and glean (pick) ears of corn after him in whose sight I shall find grace. And she said unto her, 'Go my daughter'* (Ruth 2:2). She gleaned . . . wheat not the Indian corn of America. Ruth would have gleaned from not only Boaz field, but anyone who would be friendly and permit her to glean in

their field. As it happened it was Boaz who owned the field where she worked; it was he who showed her favor. It was the custom in Israel and commanded in the law that the corners of the fields be left for the poor, and a sheaf left in the field was to remain there for them . . . (Dake's Bible).

When you reap the harvest of the land, do not reap to the very edges of your field or gather the gleanings (pickings) of your harvest. Do not go over your vineyard a second time or pick up the grapes that have fallen. Leave them for the poor and the alien. I am the LORD your God (Leviticus 19:9, 10 NIV).

Boaz was a relative, through Naomi's departed husband Elimelech, a man of great wealth. While Ruth gleaned wheat in his field, Boaz became aware of her presence and extended her favor. He instructed the men working in the field to allow extra wheat to fall on the ground so that she could pick it up. He also commanded the young men working for him not to touch her. Boaz requested Ruth to only glean in his field; he knew she would then be safe. She bowed in gratitude to this stranger who further informed her that he had heard all that she had done to help her mother-in-law. Boaz was aware of her leaving her father's house to come to a foreign land to be with Naomi.

In the Book of Ruth Chapter Three, Naomi talks to Ruth about finding security for her. She explained that Boaz would be "*winnowing barley tonight at the threshing floor.*" She then gave Ruth specific instructions to follow:

Therefore wash yourself and anoint yourself, put on your best garment and go down to the threshing floor, but do not make yourself known to the man until he

> *has finished eating and drinking. Then it shall be when he lies down, that you shall notice the place where he lies; and you shall go in, uncover his feet, and lie down; and he will tell you what you should do . . . So she went down to the threshing floor and did according to all that her mother-in-law instructed her* (Ruth 3:2-4, 6 NKJV).

Ruth was obedient to follow her mother-in-law's instructions. Naomi and Ruth's story is a beautiful narrative concerning love, trust, relationships and restoration. Sometimes it helps to have a seasoned mentor who is looking out for your welfare to assist you in reaching your God-ordained purpose.

> *Now it happened at midnight that the man was startled and turned himself, and there was a woman lying at his feet. And he said, 'Who are you?' So she answered, "I am Ruth, your maidservant. Take your maidservants under your wings, for you are a close relative* (Ruth 3:8, 9 NKJV).

Boaz tells Ruth that he knows she is a virtuous woman. He admits that he is a close relative but that there is another relative closer to Elimelech than he. It was the Jewish custom to find out if the closest relative would redeem property from the deceased, and also marry the wife of the deceased. Boaz went to the city to find the other relative; he did not procrastinate but hurriedly met with the other relative about being Naomi's kinsman redeemer: "*Then Boaz said, "On the day you buy the field from the hand of Naomi, you must also buy it from Ruth the Moabitess, the wife of the dead, to perpetuate the name of the dead through his inheritance*" (Ruth 4:5 NKJV).

The closest relative could not marry Ruth, for it would have ruined his inheritance. "*So Boaz took Ruth and she became his wife, and when he went in to her, the Lord gave her conception, and she bore a son*" (Ruth 4:13 NKJV). Their son was called Obed; he later became the father of Jesse and King David's grandfather. Naomi took the child in her bosom and nursed him. What a great ending for Naomi and Ruth who were faithful to God and to each other! God rewards the faithful; and this is a prime example of two faithful people being rewarded for their perseverance.

Ruth married Boaz and became an ancestor of Jesus the Christ. It is significant to also remember that Boaz as a kinsman redeemer was a man of great wealth, for when God restores He favors in every area of your life. The child from Boaz and Ruth's union was a blessing to Naomi and brought restoration to her in her senior years. The story of Naomi and Ruth allows others to see that you do not have to rest in your grief and loneliness; a breakout of your mess will lead you to a breakthrough into the blessed promises of recovery. Identify yourself with the One you are in covenant with for deliverance, healing, and restoration.

God wants to give you testimonies of His promises being fulfilled in your life; it is not over until He says so. God desires to turn your mourning into dancing, to give you beauty for ashes. See yourself coming out of your situation with favorable results. You have to see it and declare it before you receive it. God will do what seemingly is impossible for you. God—your exceeding great reward—will allow you to bear fruit perpetually for His Kingdom. Remember, your darkest hour very well could be just before you receive your incredible blessing!

2

IDENTITY CRISIS

Women everywhere are experiencing an identity crisis! This chapter is purposely focused more on women than men due to the many challenges women have faced, are facing today, and will encounter in the future. The female gender has been long devalued by family, society, and the church.

The family should be the first to provide love, security and protection for a child, but many families are dysfunctional—functioning outside of the role as models to love, nourish, protect, instruct, and discipline. The family should be the first line of defense for young females, as well as young males; yet it is often the place of much pain, shame and devastation. Even the church has looked upon some females with a condescending attitude, as an object to blame, shame, and condemn. Females are looking for affirmation of their identity. Though affirmation should begin in the home, it has not always been received from the male parent or, at times, even from the mother. The truth of the matter is that many females have been rejected from their mother's womb or during early childhood, and such rejection has been effective in helping to create an identity crisis.

June Hunt, author of *Counseling Through Your Bible Handbook,* shares some interesting points on identity through the following questions: "Who are you really? Do you identify yourself with your occupation: 'I'm a teacher' or with your nationality, 'I'm a German' or with your struggles, 'I'm an alcoholic'?" Hunt adds: "All of these labels do help identify us by distinguishing us one from another, but they are not primary identity. Based on the Bible, everyone on earth is identified with one of two persons—either Adam or Jesus. And the implications of whose family line you belong to are a matter of life and death—for eternity."

When someone shows partiality toward another it could possibly have a negative effect on the other person, especially if they are experiencing some identity issues. Children have a way of devaluing other children and many times the adults in their lives allow the problem to escalate. Some adults devalue their children by speaking negative words over them. Sometimes the labels they place on them can be disabling or may prompt them to feel incapacitated in some area of mental-emotional progression.

Throughout church history many church leaders continually added to women's identity crisis, especially when we speak of women called into leadership roles. Women have been rejected from entering certain leadership positions in the church. Specifically, they have been discouraged from going forth in ministerial or clergy positions, such as: bishops, pastors, superintendents, elders, deacons, and chairpersons of certain groups. Some Scriptures have been taken out of context in an effort to prove that women are suppose to be silent in the church and are not to usurp authority over a man.

In most churches women make up the majority of the congregation. It has been proven, over and over again, that it has been an acceptable practice for women to lead the choir, supervise the nursery, head up the children's group, and direct kitchen affairs. Even though women have always engaged in these activities to help the church, some have known there is a higher calling on their lives; therefore, they need someone to affirm them or help them identify their purpose in ministry. Release the women while they are under your leadership, spiritual leaders; allow God to guide them in reaching their potential. Life is meaningless if a person does not discover their purpose!

Myles Monroe in *Releasing Your Potential* emphasizes that many have died without reaching their potential. Addressing the topic, "The Abortion of Ability," he cites the words of Sir Winston Churchill: "The price of greatness is responsibility." Dr. Monroe further illustrates, "The graveyards are full of great men and women who never became great because they did not give their ability responsibility. This untapped ability is called potential. Each of us comes into the world pregnant with unlimited potential . . . Unless we expose, during the course of our lives, all that God placed within us for the good of mankind, our potential will be aborted."

Women who have not been accepted in leadership positions have a tendency to devalue other women who are leaders. A spirit of jealousy exists that tries to keep women separated; this spirit is alive and active and can be disabling to women trying to reach their potential. Women are many times divided by small, insignificant things; and some will not support other women if they believe their assistance will be effective in helping others move in their purpose. We are experiencing this situation at the present time in our ministry—evidenced by a pulling back or by assistance with such carelessness that demonstrates a will to mess things up. When a sister is down there should be other sisters—and brothers—willing to undergird her in prayer . . . to support and to encourage her on the journey.

I want to emphasize how the spirit of jealousy works: First, it is a manifestation of the flesh. The Greek word for flesh is *sarx*—identifying the body, the external, which is frail, passionate, and carnal minded; it is the human aspect of a person. King Saul became very jealous of young David, after he, Saul, had been chosen by the people (flesh) to be king over God's people. The people wanted a leader—a king—to lead them, rather than continuing to be led by God. Saul was the people's choice, not God's choice.

Initially, King Saul chose David to be his armor bearer. Then he also set him over the men of war as their captain, so that David could not return again to his father to tend sheep. Saul loved David at first but later became extremely jealous of him. When Saul fell into disobedience to God, David was chosen by God to be the next king. David did not walk immediately into his divine purpose as God's chosen; it was years before he actually took the kingship. Saul ruled for forty years over Israel.

After David's victory over the Philistines, the women from all the cities of Israel came out singing and dancing as they met King Saul in celebration. The women answered one another as they played, saying:

> *Saul hath slain his thousands and David his ten thousands. And Saul was very wroth...the saying displeased him; and he said, They have ascribed unto David ten thousands and to me they have ascribed*

but thousands: and what can he have more but the kingdom? (1 Samuel18:7, 8).

Saul feared that if David continued to be successful and prosper in all that he put his hands to, he would soon have his kingship; therefore, Saul planned ways to prevent losing the kingdom to David. His jealousy began with fear of another advancing in his efforts and others praising him for his achievements. The evil spirit that God permitted to come upon King Saul, after he disobeyed God, was the cause of such jealous hatred toward David.

As you can see, jealousy is an evil spirit that will eventually destroy relationships, break up marriages, divide homes, bring stagnation to churches, infect workplaces, and shut down marketplaces. This evil spirit responsible for Saul's jealousy of David was a recurring spirit; it caused the king to make many attempts to kill David. Altogether, twenty-one attempts were made on David's life due to Saul's outrageous jealousy; but the king was not successful in carrying out his evil plans. God had chosen David to be King Saul's successor.

As a pastor, I have had women come into the church to bring confusion, strife, and division due to a jealous spirit. Women in leadership, who are plagued by this spirit, will sometimes leave a ministry without warning, in order to disrupt that ministry's vision. Admittedly, such practice hinders but cannot stop the plan of God for His work. It is amazing how some can leave a ministry offended for no justifiable reason; but God will send in others who are grateful to help fulfill the vision.

There is a competitive spirit among some women that suggests, "I can do it better than you." During our "God's

Anointed Annual Women Conference" in September 2010, Pastor Kathy Goodwin, of Coke Memorial United Methodist Church in Louisville, Kentucky, served as a guest speaker. Her focus, "Women in Authority and Women under Authority?" emphasized how some women are jealous of other women in leadership, thus competing for position or recognition. She compared their actions to that of a cheerleader who observes another cheerleader kicking, then determines, "I'm going to out kick you during this game." Some women try to compete with other women even in the church—and it should not be. There is so much to be done in the Kingdom of God; competition is not an option. In a secular game only one team can win, but in Christ all believers win because we are one in Him.

Remember when Adam and Eve were seduced by the serpent into believing they could be like God? Genesis Chapter 3 records Eve's encounter with the serpent:

> *Now the serpent was more subtle than any beast of the field which the Lord God had made. And he said unto the woman, Yea, hath God said, Ye shall not eat of every tree of the garden? And the woman said unto the serpent, We may eat of the fruit of the trees of the garden; but of the fruit of the tree which is in the midst of the garden, God hath said, ye shall not eat of it, neither shall you touch it, lest you die. And the serpent said unto the woman, Ye shall not surely die. For God doth know that in the day ye eat thereof, then your eyes shall be opened, and ye shall be as gods, knowing good and evil* (Genesis 3:1-5).

A quest to be like God caused Eve to take fruit from the tree God had forbidden Adam and Eve to eat of. Could this be the beginning of the spirit to compete with someone more advanced? "*And when the woman saw that the tree was good for food, and that it was pleasant to the eyes, and a tree to be desired to make one wise; she took of the fruit thereof, and did eat, and gave also unto her husband with her, and he did eat*" (Genesis 3:6).

Can you now envision the root of jealousy and competition? Satan as the anointed Cherub was thrown out of Heaven when he strategized to dethrone God in his mind. Satan wanted to compete with God, but he only won one-third of the angels when he rebelled against Him. Jealousy and competition are works of the flesh and the master mind behind these self-willed deeds is the devil, our adversary, our enemy. Eve was created in perfect harmony with God's mind and heart and identified as *woman* for she came out of *ma*n Adam. Eve lost her perfect identity when she sinned with Adam and hid what God had created to be beautiful.

Why is it critical to know your identity? It becomes a crisis when a lack of identity is instrumental in influencing you to abort your purpose. Women are crucial to the eternal plan of God in birthing forth others to fulfill their purpose while on earth. Some women have determined they are of little value and worth because they have not discovered who they are in the Kingdom of God. This is why we need more mentors; oftentimes, it takes a female mentor to identify the struggles and assist in aiding another female to discover her purpose. When you have been devalued from birth or never affirmed positively during your childhood, you may assume that this is the way of life. Unless someone comes into your life to change your perspective and mentor you out of your wounded state, you have little reason to expect anything else. You may find yourself in one critical situation after another.

Sometimes, a child may be rejected from the mother's womb because the timing for pregnancy was not appropriate, or the gender was not what the parents expected or hoped. As an embryo is developing, it is able to experience the "coldness" and aloof attitude of the parent. A child developing within the womb of a parent who loves him or her will have a different attitude than one whose parent does not love that child. Needless crying as an infant may be a psychological response to parental rejection.

During my first pregnancy I cried often because I felt alone and rejected by the person who partnered with me in the conception of my child. I was eighteen when conception took place, and therefore, young, naïve, and confused. I did not feel good about myself nor about the child growing in my womb; fear and shamed plagued me because I was pregnant and unmarried. It is important to love your child while in the womb because your emotions do have an impact on their well-being.

It has been well documented how drugs, alcohol, cigarettes, and other harmful things ingested in the body during pregnancy affect the fetus. It is the same with a woman whose emotional state is not well balanced. Fear, shame, anger, rejection, and hurt can be experienced while in the womb. The opposite of rejection is love, acceptance, and security. Fortunately, these too can penetrate and saturate the inner most being of your child. Both negative and positive emotions have a direct influence on your fetus, and ultimately on your child when he or she is born.

Rejection is a negative force that causes a person to experience alienation and low self-worth. Many females have been rejected when it was revealed that a male was not in the womb, or this was discovered immediately after birth.

I have had the opportunity to speak with certain women who rejected their child upon discovering they were pregnant, especially some single parents. Some single, female parents rejected their child during pregnancy, but loved him or her immediately upon seeing their baby. One mother told me that she always tells her daughter she loves her, to lessen the chance of her feeling rejected, because she initially rejected her daughter from the womb.

Some females have been reared in homes where the parent(s) treated them as one would treat a male child. They may have dressed or do occasionally dress their child with clothes more suitable for a male. They may also engage her in rough play or sports, and make her do work around the home that is more appropriate for the male gender. Some also exhibit disappointment when a female is their first born—just another of a few negative points of view as to why some women develop an identity crisis.

Seeking to discover who you are in a society that perpetuates male chauvinism can be very challenging, which is why it is so important to have spiritual mentors to help you reclaim God's purpose for your life. You are not a mistake; there is a purpose for you being here on earth, and God has the final say about your life. When God created male and female, He declared everything He made was good. When God could not swear by anyone greater, He swore by Himself.

The New Revised Standard Version Bible of Genesis 1:26-30 states:

> *So God created humankind in His image, in the image of God He created them; male and female He created them. God blessed them, and God said to them, Be*

fruitful and multiply, and fill the earth and subdue it; and have dominion over the fish of the sea and over the birds of the air and over every living thing that moves upon the earth. God said, See, I have given you every plant yielding seed that is upon the face of all the earth, and every tree with seed in its fruit; you shall have them for food. And to every beast of the earth and to ever bird of the air and to everything that creeps on the earth, everything that has the breath of life, I have given every green plant for food. And it was so.

Humankind is not a term found in the Bible, but the term *man* is used numerous times in reference to male and female. Most Bibles are written using exclusive language and, therefore, are not particularly inclusive when it comes to females. *The New Revised Standard Version* utilizes inclusive language; thus, some female readers prefer using it, to avoid exclusivity.

A belief exists among some female scholars that the Bible is written addressing the male with a tendency to oppress the female. Dr. Maisha Handy, Assistant Professor of Christian Education at the Interdenominational Theological Center, Atlanta, Georgia, addresses this belief in an article published in the seminary's journal titled "Fighting the Matrix: Toward A Womanist Pedagogy for the Black Church." Similarly, Dr. Jacquelyn Grant, a Calloway Professor of Theology at the same seminary, describes females as being oppressed threefold: through sexism, racism, and classism. There are some individuals and some systems that still oppress particular ethnic groups, certain classes, and demonstrate gender prejudice. Certain traditions have practiced or promoted segregation among the genders for centuries; but, of course, we know that in God's Kingdom there is neither *male* nor *female:*

"There is neither Jew nor Greek, there is neither slave nor free; there is neither male nor female for ye are one in Christ Jesus. And if you be Christ's, then you are Abraham's seed, and heirs according to the promise" (Galatians 3:28, 29).

Donald K. McKim states, in *Westminster Dictionary of Theological Terms,* "Patriarchal is a term used for a particular cultural attitude of those men whose way of acting toward women is oppressive, especially in their use of power. It is male domination over every aspect of women's existence—political, economic, social, sexual, religious, and various other ways." During the fall of 1999, as a student at the Louisville Presbyterian Theological Seminary and while taking a theology course, I was introduced to inclusive language. It was foreign to me. Earlier in 1991, I had begun the graduate program at Southern Baptist Theological Seminary, and during my tenure there inclusive language was not a part of the curriculum, nor would be. It became evident after its new president was sworn in and proceeded to make changes that women, as preachers and teachers, were out of place in the seminary environment of Southern Baptist. Some professors, who were married, left Southern Baptist to seek employment elsewhere; they sought an environment that was more conducive to accepting both male and female. Several male professors who were married could not continue to teach in an institution that would no longer affirm women in ministry.

Women have been oppressed for centuries. This became most evident to me when I visited a Bible College in Louisville during the nineties and was told by staff there that female students were not permitted to take preaching courses; they were for men only. It was the consensus of the Bible College staff and faculty that women were not called by God to preach. Women, however, have been called to preach, teach, prophesy, and lead others since the foundation of the earth.

I do not know what happened in the first created earth which was ruled by Lucifer the Archangel of worship; but after the second creation, male and female were created equal. When God created Adam and Eve, He established equal rights between them over the rest of God's creation. They were in a higher position to have dominion over other created things because they were created in the image of God. Adam ruled before God brought forth a beautiful woman to be by his side; for he was not whole without *woman.* God saw that he needed a helper and supplied that need. With all God had put under his authority, God knew it was not good for *man* to be alone: Adam needed someone comparable to him, yet different, for the purpose of procreation.

God saw that Adam was lonely, so He made Adam a helpmeet, an aide—someone to assist him. Such is the case with the Holy Spirit, our Comforter, our Helper—the Greek *paraklētŏs.* He is called alongside of us to be our Comforter, Aide, Intercessor, Consoler or Advocate.

I must emphasize here the nature of Creator God or *Elohim,* the Father, the Son and the Holy Spirit. God created male and female and placed *them* over His earthly creation. Adam was given the earth to rule over; however, God saw that he was lonely and needed a helper. The woman was to assist the man in having dominion over God's created order; she was not to be a 'door mat' or to be controlled by man, for they were to share equally as partners. God is concerned about your every need being met; therefore, God gives you the desires of your heart. Because sin had not yet entered into the heart of humankind, Adam was in the perfect will of God, to receive anything from the Creator.

The creation story, as told in Genesis Chapters 1-2, records how God recreated the earth and formed humankind in His likeness and image. It describes how Adam and Eve walked in the presence of God, and that they communed with Him daily. They were openly exposed to God and were without shame, for they shared in the perfect order of God's creation. God declared that everything created by Him was good.

After the fall in the Garden of Eden (Genesis Chapter 3), Adam and Eve hid themselves from God and attempted to cover their nakedness with fig leaves. Eve's subtle seduction via the serpent was a way to test God concerning the fruit that was not to be eaten. Eve took of the fruit and gave it to her mate. Remember, they were equal partners, who did not have an identity crisis before they disobeyed God; so when she offered the forbidden fruit to her husband, he took of it. There had never been before a need for domination and control over another person. Being equal partners, they were both equally driven from the Garden of Eden, from the presence of God—forbidden to ever enter again. God showed no partiality in judging them. Eve lost her place of equality after the fall, but gained it back through Christ.

After Adam and Eve sinned against God, they lost their place of authority over the earthly realm. The fall of humanity from the grace and glory of God subjected the man and woman to suffer, and to eventually die. They were created to live perpetually or eternally if they had continued to obey God. This was a big fall for humankind, and all of humanity has suffered ever since. After the fall humanity suffered from an identity crisis, that is, all those born from the loins of Adam were identified with Adam. Since the fall, the identity of those who believe has been regained through accepting the Second Adam, Christ. After the fall women were forced to give birth through pain and sorrow, and to suffer through a whole new way of sustaining life—by the sweat of man's face.

Women have been accused of having a "Jezebel spirit" partly because Eve was blamed for seducing Adam into eating the fruit. Let me enlightened you a little bit about the character of Jezebel. She was a woman in the Bible who was despised because of her destructive nature of licentious, which means sexually unrestrained nature. She was a person who was devoted to sensual pleasures, with all the cheap showy arts of a wanton woman. She was devoted to having those under her rulership worship the gods of Baal and Ashtoreth. She was married to Ahab a weak, spineless king who was over Northern Israel; she led him to defy the God of Israel and worship these false gods. He allowed her to exercise authority over him and his domain. She was arrogant, proud, ambitious, seductive, wicked, strong-minded, savage, relentless, overbearing domineering, and persuasive in all of her wrongly directed deeds. She was actually a person who died in her own filth. Eve on the other hand was deceived and her husband was deceived by their own desire to test God's Word. How will you tie this to the biblical Jezebel?]

Many times women in the church have been labeled with a Jezebel calling; the first time they tried to exercise their gifts they were labeled as having the spirit of Jezebel. At other times it is misused when there are wives in the church who believe certain women are lusting after their husband, and the one being accused is labeled "Jezebel." After reading about her character it will be hard to find a match for this character. —The Jezebel that existed in 1 Kings was not a believer in the God of Israel, this is the reason she seduced her husband King Ahab, and the people under his jurisdiction to worship false gods. We have to guard against putting false labels on folk.

I want to reemphasize that Adam and Eve were equal in nature, attributes, intellect, mind, will, class, emotions, and body, though not reproductive organs. *Woman* was taken out of *Man* and they both do have some of the same hormones, but God made them male and female, for the sake of procreation. The fall of Adam and Eve, which occurred over six thousand years ago, has been under the blood of Jesus for over two thousand years; Christ came as our Advocate to help us regain our identity. Women are not to be low-class citizens, so-called door mats, punching bags, slaves, bondwomen, or victims under abuse by others. Women are liberated due to the Calvary experience!

Sadly, many religious organizations have been instrumental in oppressing women to the degree of humiliation, shame and fear. Wounded women need to be delivered and healed on the inside from such oppression. Yet deliverance is hindered due to religious traditions and the worship of false, inanimate gods. When you cannot make a decision for yourself, you are in bondage. The example of some women having to wear hot clothes covering everything but their eyes in certain male-dominated cultures is one sign of oppression suffered by women. This is not the will of the true and living God for them. The inability of some who cannot correct their children or help in making decisions about their home because of fear is a form of spousal abuse. Some men take being head of the household too far: When they oppress or abuse their mate, the family structure is destroyed. To be set free in your mind, you must discover your purpose. You were created in the likeness and image of God our Creator; you are wonderfully and beautifully made and are not to be trampled on. Cry out to the Lord Jesus Christ day and night; He will come to your aid!

In 1988 God called me into ministry while I was engaged in the "ministry of helps" at a local Baptist church in the city of Louisville, Kentucky. At that time, I was president of the church choir. As long as I was a lay person, it was acceptable for me to lead worship from the pulpit, but the day I acknowledged my call into the ministry of the Word, the attitude of some church leaders changed toward me: I was told (repeating verbatim), "You better not go into that pulpit." In other words, it was not acceptable for me to lead the church into worship on Sunday mornings standing behind the podium as previously done: "Now that you say God has called you into the ministry, we do not believe it. We do not believe God call women to preach, so stay out of the pulpit." Women have been oppressed for centuries trying to do the work of the Kingdom; this oppression is not a new thing, but is often done in subtle ways.

Females who are molested or raped, which is, non-consensual, forced sexual intercourse are oppressed by their aggressor. I have met numerous females who were molested by males which, of course, had a traumatic influence on these women: Some find it difficult to get involved in a relationship with someone of the opposite sex because of past trauma. Some have become promiscuous among men. Others have resorted to engaging in relationships of intimacy with someone of the same sex. Traumatic effects come out of having experienced sexual encounters at the hand of someone who was suppose to protect . . . as a father, grandfather, brother or uncle. Because of sexual abuse, some women have *subverted* or *devalued* the whole meaning of sexual intimacy the way God intended it to occur—between husband and wife. Instead of experiencing sexual intimacy in marriage with someone who loves God, loves her as a woman, and loves himself, she has been made to feel ashamed, fearful, angry, unclean, defiled, helpless and without control, or freedom of choice. Some have been made to feel as if totally stripped of dignity, integrity, and identity. Counseling—godly counseling—needs to be there for their total recovery. Women, find someone you trust to help you with your deliverance and healing and cry out to the Lord God for help during your deliverance!

Many females have been robbed of their virginity... some have not had one person in whom they could trust and confide in. To carry such a burden into adulthood has to be a lonely journey. Girls have been told, "Don't rock the boat" or "Keep it within the family" or "Don't tell anyone; they will take you away from me." Some female children or adolescents taken out of their home have sustained sexual, emotional, and physical abuse while in foster homes. There does not seem to be a major or widespread concern about the short-term or long-term effects on these innocent and abused children.

Withholding from someone financially when it is in your power to give and you are obligated to provide support is another form of oppression. I had a young woman inform me about how her husband oppressed her financially by withholding necessary funds for daily living. She finally separated from him. As mentioned previously, females are not always treated with the same kind of respect when it comes to getting leadership positions. Sometimes the pay scale for females is lower than that for males, even for the same position. Financial discrimination is another way of devaluing females. To overcome the situation, one must trust God and "speak those things that are not as though they were," as stated in Romans 4:17.

I am so grateful and must re-emphasize that there is neither male nor female in Christ; we are one in Him. When God created *man* He was referring to all humanity: *"Adam,"* the Hebrew word for *man* means *human being*. We humans find our identity in Christ. The blood of Jesus, shed for removal of our sins, allows believers in Jesus the Christ to be adopted into the family of God, which also includes identifying with Christ (the Anointed One). It does not matter what we have had to endure in life; our purpose is in Him and so is ultimately our identity. Press toward the prize which is Christ Jesus because it is He who liberates us from all forms of oppression! Most importantly, you must discover who you are in the Kingdom of God and see yourself through the eyes of Christ.

3

AVOID THE GRASSHOPPER MENTALITY: Low Self Esteem

One of the greatest deliverances in the history of the Hebrew Bible took place when God used Moses to deliver the Israelites from Egyptian bondage. The account is recorded in Exodus Chapter 14. It was one of the largest supernatural deliverances in the Scriptures. The new king of Egypt did not know the history of the Hebrews or Israelites and saw them as a threat to his kingdom. Fear of them growing numerically and possibly joining with other enemies during wartime caused Pharaoh to put the children of God in slavery, with taskmasters overseeing them. With this new Pharaoh the Israelites had to endure forced labor, oppression, domination, control, even the slaying of all Hebrew newborn males born during the time of Moses' birth. God prepared a leader that was well equipped to deliver His children from this Egyptian king.

God will always raise or set up and mobilize a general to execute His will and plan whenever there is a major assignment to be done. That general must be someone who will sacrifice everything to obey God; someone who will therefore yield to the adequate preparation that is necessary. Generals need time for their character to be developed and they need to acquire patience to wait on God during the training process. Potential leaders need to be equipped, so God personally taught Moses and then raised up his brother Aaron as a mentor. Moses' sister Miriam and father-in-law Jethro were also among those added to his support team.

God, in His infinite wisdom, takes the foolish things of this world to confound the wise. In other words, God chooses weak, insignificant things to shame those things that are mighty, according to 1 Corinthians 1:27. Moses had a speech impediment, which caused him to stutter and lack self confidence. Furthermore, Moses exhibited a strong temper and in anger lashed out and killed an Egyptian to protect a fellow Hebrew. Fearing the backlash, Moses ran into the wilderness for his life; but God called him out of hiding to be a general over His army.

The Israelites had been slaves for over four hundred years; they received only the bare necessities for their survival. God, in His omnipotence, gave them the wealth of Egypt within a twenty-four hour period. One moment of favor from God can establish a person, a business, a ministry, or some other work for a lifetime. One moment of favor from God will remove every hindrance or stumbling block to see a vision through to fruition. It may tarry, but wait on the vision to be fulfilled; it will come to pass:

> *Write the vision and make it plain that he may run who reads it, for the vision is yet for an appointed time; but at the end it will speak and it will not lie.*

> *Though it tarries, wait for it, because it will surely come to pass* (Habakkuk 2:2, 3 NKJV).

When the Lord remembered his promises to Abraham, Isaac, and Jacob, He had to abide by the covenant made to them. Our God is a covenant keeper; He will not break His covenant made to His believers. According to Genesis 17:1, God made a covenant with Abram when he was ninety-nine years old. The Lord asked Abram to walk before Him and be perfect, that is, his heart was to be wholly and sincerely devoted to God:

> *And I will make my covenant (solemn pledge) between me and you and will multiply you exceedingly. Then Abram fell on his face, and God said to him, As for me, behold, My covenant (solemn pledge) is with you, and you shall be a father of many nations. Nor shall your name any longer be Abram [high, exalted father], but your name shall be Abraham [father of a multitude], for I have made you the father of many nations* (Genesis 17:2-5 AMP).

The Hebrew word here for covenant is *beriyth,* which means compact, league, or confederacy. Covenant also means mutual agreement.

God had to raise up a leader to deliver the Israelites out of Egyptian bondage because of the covenant He had established with Abraham. Moses was that chosen leader. The assignment was so great. Moses began to make excuses concerning his incompetence. It was not easy for Moses, who had to go back to the same Egyptian leaders he had been raised under and demand that they let God's people go. Freedom had to come so that the Israelites could worship God the way God ordained and in the place God designated. This is another example of taking the foolish things to confound the wise. When given an assignment by the Lord, there is going to be some preparation time; wait on it. Moses had to be purged of Egyptian culture, fear, dread, doubt, and of making excuses about his inarticulate speech in order to go forth. He had some low self-esteem issues with his new assignment. As the prince of Egypt Moses would have succeeded there—yet that was not his purpose for being born.

Moses ran for his life when it was known that he had killed an Egyptian to protect a Hebrew slave; he fled Egypt into Midian. Now God was asking him to go back and to command that the Israelites be released from bondage to worship Him. Moses more than likely feared returning to Egypt, but God was saying, "Go, tell Pharaoh to let my people go." When Moses returned to Egypt, God did miracles through the hands of Moses, but Pharaoh was not impressed. God sent plagues, but Pharaoh would not release the Israelites. The tenth plague brought devastation to Egypt; it was responsible for the death of all the firstborn males of Egypt. With it God's plan was successfully executed; His children were freed from slavery. Pharaoh was broken because his only son died in the plague; thus, he surrendered and released the Israelites.

Remember, an earlier Pharaoh tried to destroy all the Israelite male babies during the time when Moses was born. Moses' mother saw that he was a special child and hid him, thereby sparing his life. This same curse came back upon the Egyptians; the death angel swept through Egypt and destroyed every firstborn male, including Pharaoh's son. "*Do not be deceived, God is not mocked; for whatever a man sows, that he will also reap*" (Galatians 6:7). The Egyptians did reap what they had previously sown.

God gave specific orders for Moses to follow in order for the Israelites to exit Egypt safely. The homes of the Israelites had to be marked with blood; this action was so God's chosen people would avoid the death plague that would pass through. God said to Moses:

> *For I will pass through the land of Egypt on that night, and will strike all the firstborn in the land of Egypt, both male and beast, and against the gods of Egypt I will execute judgment. I am the Lord. Now the blood shall be a sign for you on the houses where you are, and when I see the blood, I will pass over you. The plague shall not be on you to destroy you when I strike the land of Egypt* (Exodus 12:12, 13NKJV).

God instituted *Passover* as a memorial for every generation to keep; a feast to the Lord in remembrance of that great day when God delivered the Israelites.

The Israelites left Egypt suddenly in obedience to God, and with great wealth. They were to reap what they had sown: the Israelites had built Egypt's great cities with forced labor, blood, sweat, and tears, and they had only received the bare necessities to sustain their lives. God did not allow them to leave Egypt financially destitute or feeble in their bodies. They asked for wealth from the Egyptians and received their request. One day of favor from the Lord can turn your whole life around!

Moses and the Israelites left Egypt but were soon pursued by Pharaoh and his army. God hardened Pharaoh's heart so that he would pursue the Israelites to seek revenge. Moses and the Israelites found themselves caught between the Red Sea and the enemy's army. God had to show Himself mighty and strong before a people who were fearful of their enemy's approaching forces.

> *Then Moses stretched out his hand over the sea; and the LORD caused the sea to go back by a strong east wind all that night, and made the sea into dry land, and the waters were divided. So the children of Israel went into the midst of the sea on the dry ground, and the waters were a wall to them on their right hand and on their left* (Exodus14:21, 22 NKJV).

What an awesome deliverance by the mighty hand of God! That one act of God should have encouraged the Israelites to trust in Him to meet all their other needs. This was also a testimony of Moses' continual confidence and maturity in God. Moses did not waiver in God's divine enablement to see them through this ordeal.

John C. Maxwell, author of *The Maxwell Leadership Bible*, states, "The approach of the Egyptian army terrified the Israelites, and they placed heavy pressure on Moses to handle this crisis. Moses didn't panic, since he had seen the power of God's handiwork. Instead, he exuded both poise and peace, winning for himself great credibility as a leader." Maxwell goes on to state that "Moses gained credibility through the law of buy-in by four qualities. He projected calm instead of craziness, confidence instead of cowardice, clarity instead of confusion, and competence instead of clumsiness. He became the nation's go to leader through this one incident."

In spite of their breakthrough and deliverance from Egyptian bondage, the Israelites were never able to come into their destiny as the chosen people of God. They were wounded from years of abuse; they suffered from low self esteem, not believing in themselves. Only two spies out of twelve were able to go into the land of promise—Joshua and Caleb. It is possible for some people to never experience the favor of God in their personal lives, in the area of inner healing; they are dominated by fear, rejection, low self-worth, and defeatism. The Israelites were fearful of the giants in Canaan; the thought of trying to possess the land with these enormous people present was horrifying to them. In other words, they became in their sight what they believed about themselves. They believed they were like grasshoppers in their mind, so they failed to take the promise land because of fear of losing the battle against the giants. They did not trust God, their leader, nor themselves to go up against the giants. "*For as he thinks in his heart, so is he*" (Proverbs 23:7a).

One Hebrew word for heart is *labe* which usually refers to some aspect of the immaterial, inner self. The Strong's Concordance gives us the Hebrew meaning for *labe: "the heart is considered to be the seat of one's inner nature as well as one of its components. It can be used to define a specific aspect of the personality, the mind, the will, and the emotions; it alludes to the inside or middle.*" The Israelites suffered from heart issues that would later become problematic to the point of stagnating them in a major cycle of their life span. In other words, the Israelites not only needed deliverance, they needed healing from past memories, thoughts, and emotions.

They trusted God only as long as they could see Him moving on their behalf; their generation was not born in an environment motivated by trust. For hundreds of years, they were a people told what to do . . . how to do . . . where to do . . . when to do . . . and why it needed to be done. The Israelites were punished harshly when they did not follow the strict guidelines of their slave masters. Familiarity with

Egypt and its harsh treatments, rendered by Pharaoh's slave masters, was more tolerable to them than being free in an unfamiliar place. God's people had issues learning to trust a God they could not see. Is that your issue today? Until we do see Him face to face we as believers walk by faith, which is the confidence we have in His Word, that He is who He says He is. We see all the evidence of a true and living God through our daily lives, throughout the earth as we look at: hills, mountains, birds, flowers, and from the peace we experience even during a time of economic hardship, political-social oppression.

The Israelites were a wounded nation of people and moving them out of their situation did not necessarily bring healing and restoration. They longed to return to what was familiar, rather than moving forward into the promise. Many times in an abusive situation, the abused will return to what has been familiar to them, because they are fearful of the unknown. Some who have been abused will ask, "How am I to make it alone? Where will I find a place to live? Who will assist me to pay the bills?" Sadly, even after leaving the person who is abusive, the abused sometimes return; they lack vision to see how they might survive in a different setting.

The Israelites were supernaturally released from Pharaoh as slaves but never recovered from the slave mentality. *Webster's New World Dictionary* defines the word "slave" as meaning "bondsman, bondservant, bondwoman . . . victim of tyranny . . . human being who is owned as property by another, or one dominated by another's influence." The Israelites had been oppressed for over four hundred years; each generation over that period of time had suffered spiritual, emotional, mental, physical and economic oppression. The four hundred years date back from Isaacs's confirmation as the heir and seed of Abraham, until they were released from Egypt. God's people cried out to God to be delivered by reason of their oppression, and God heard them! Physically they left Egypt, but a spiritual transformation did not occur; therefore, they were disabled in their transition into the Promise Land.

When Moses was called to be the deliverer of the Israelites, he did not realize the depth of his assignment. God had to assure Moses of His identity because some incredible events were going to take place in his ministry. He knew Moses would need to know who it was that had called him to such a task, and who was going to see him through to its assigned end. After God identified Himself as the God of Moses' father, the God of Abraham, the God of Isaac, and the God of Jacob, He then revealed to Moses the purpose for his being called. This was a most unusual way of God presenting Himself to someone He summoned to do a work for Him—He got Moses' attention through a burning bush, a bush that was not being consumed. Exodus 3:7-10 records the event:

> *And the Lord said, "I have surely seen the oppression of My people who are in Egypt, and have heard their cry because of their taskmasters, for I know their sorrows. So I have come down to deliver them out of the hand of the Egyptians, and to bring them up from that land to a good and large land, to a land flowing with milk and honey, to the place of the Canaanites and the Hittites and the Amorites and the Perizzites and the Hivites and the Jebusites. Now therefore, behold, the cry of the children of Israel has come to Me, and I have also seen the oppression with which the Egyptians oppressed them. "Come now therefore, and I will send you to Pharaoh that you may*

> *bring My people, the children of Israel, out of Egypt* (NKJV).

This passage of scripture is encouraging even for us today. God does hear and He will answer you. It may seem like a long time, but wait. His ears are not so dull He cannot hear. Something is being processed in you during the waiting period. We may not understand it at the time, but good will come out of what we release to Him to rectify. Moses was puzzled or perplexed about the call. He had been raised up in the Egyptian culture under Pharaoh and groomed to be the prince of Egypt; and he was familiar with worshipping many gods as was the culture of the Egyptians. Although reared from infancy by the Egyptian ruler's sister, he was indeed a Hebrew by ethnicity. Moses was going through some identity issues. God had to inform him that he had been called and chosen to be a deliverer for His people. The God of creation, the God of Abraham, Isaac, and Jacob had to encourage Moses in His identity as God the Father. Moses needed reassurance:

> *But Moses said to God, "Who am I that I should go to Pharaoh and that I should bring the children of Israel out of Egypt?" So He said, "I will certainly be with you. And this shall be a sign to you that I have sent you; When you have brought the people out of Egypt, you shall serve God on this mountain* (Exodus 3:11,12 NKJV).

The designated place of worship was Mount Sinai, called "the mountain of God" or "the mount of the Lord." *Horeb* is often referred to as *Sinai* according to the *Holman Bible Dictionary.*

Idolatry is an issue for all cultures who practice other religions, rather than Christianity. They have to see the god they serve; there must be some visible image of their gods, such as in Buddhism and Hinduism. People want to touch, see, and feel who and what they worship. Idol worshipers are not concerned about a god who answers when they call, or one who stands for justice and truth. They serve many gods; so if one god does not answer, they can call upon another god who they believe will intervene in their situation to bring relief.

Moses left the Israelites to go up on the mountain to commune with God. The Israelites felt as if Moses had deserted them; therefore, they pressured Aaron, Moses' brother the priest, into constructing their own god, a golden calf, and began to worship the golden calf in Moses' absence. The Egyptian culture worshiped idol gods; so the Israelites reverted to what they had seen practiced for over four hundred years.

They practiced idolatry while Moses was in the presence of the Lord receiving instructions for the *church* he was called to pastor. As Moses was coming down from the mountain, he could hear the party going on; and he was stunned! His brother Aaron, the priest, was in charge but had given in to the people's demands, fears and frustrations. Satan comes to frustrate the plans of God; you have to be settled in your commitment to follow God; otherwise, you may yield to temptation to oppose Him. Believers in Christ cannot waiver in their faith when tempted, because temptation will always come! We will be tempted with the lust of the flesh, the lust of the eyes, and the pride of life, just as Adam, Eve, and Jesus were tempted. The only difference, Adam and Eve sinned—Jesus did not. The Lord has made a way of escape for every person, but we have to be willing to step out into the unfamiliar, and to reject the demands made on us.

Moses was angry when he saw the church practicing idol worship. One of the reasons God brought them out of Egypt was to settle them in a place God had chosen to worship Him. Moses' anger, or righteous indignation, flared up when he saw the people acting like the folk in Egypt. He threw down the tables with the Ten Commandments written on them by God, and rebuked their foolishness for engaging in such practice. It had taken forty years after Moses left Egypt to be delivered from the Egyptian culture, so that God could use him. Now the people had been brought out of Egypt but Egyptian culture was still in them. The Israelites could not identify with the God of Abraham, Isaac, and Jacob; and they suddenly forgot their deliverance from the Egyptian army, and how they had crossed the Red Sea on dry land. They needed deliverance and inner healing, which would only come through believing God and the miracles He had performed for them. They had to trust God and God's chosen leader. The Holy Spirit had not yet come to dwell in believers; but He was with them. They would have to trust a God they could not see.

God established his covenant or contract with the Israelite congregation by giving Moses laws by which the people would be governed. He commanded the people: "*You shall be holy, for I the Lord your God am holy*" (Leviticus 19:2). Worship was established according to God's design. Worship was what God expected from His chosen people then, even as He expects from us today. Once you have an encounter with the Almighty God, you begin to identity with Him and His will for your life. Those who dwell in the flesh will never get to that place. God has to separate you from what you have always identified with in order to establish your true identity and purpose.

Moses accepted his God-given identity and was fulfilling his purpose. He served the people from morning till late evening as a judge, pastor, and priest. Jethro, priest of Midian and Moses' father-in-law, came to the campsite while the Israelites were wandering in the wilderness. He saw the responsibility that was on Moses, because he observed Moses judging the people from morning till night. Jethro then instructed Moses in a more effective way to take care of the congregation's needs, keep his sanity, and be able to endure. He had Moses to appoint honorable, teachable, trustworthy men to assist him in overseeing the people. The people never were delivered from their old mindset; this is the reason they remained in the wilderness for forty years. You can be set free from one form of bondage and still remain oppressed by some other influence. The generation that Moses led in the wilderness had to die… they could not see themselves obtaining the promises God ordained for them.

Moses was committed to his call but he was not appreciated by the congregation. This attitude is still true in the twenty-first century church. Many spiritual leaders are worshipers and are dedicated to the work to which God has called them, but meet continual opposition and challenges from the people being served. It is important for you to know you have been called to the office you occupy; otherwise, you will not stay encouraged to endure. Make sure of your calling! Moses had to be reassured during his tedious journey. Speaking from sixteen years of experience as a pastor, a person in that office may not always be appreciated, but you cannot quit when situations seem to overwhelm you. This is the time you need to go to the secret place, only you and the Holy Spirit. He will lead you to a place of rest, peace and comfort to stay encouraged while fulfilling the call.

The congregation rebelled against Moses, but God used him as a powerful intercessor. An intercessor is one who stands in the gap for another. Moses had to fall on his face many times and cry out to God to save His people, rather than destroy them for their rebellion. At one point in the journey, Aaron, his priestly brother, as well as his sister Miriam—also a minister—complained against God's servant. Can you imagine a church body of two to three million complaining against you? God allowed the Israelites' journey to be lengthy so that they could be disciplined. God always came through with what was necessary to sustain them; their clothes and shoes never wore out, neither was there sickness in their body. Yet instead of their faith getting stronger and settling their confidence in His provisions, God's people continued to waiver.

They needed deliverance and healing before they could proceed with the vision. They traveled and camped at different sites as God guided them with a cloud by day and fire by night. Moses did not forget the promises God made to Abraham, Isaac, and Jacob, knowing they applied to each generation in succession. God promised to bring them to a land flowing with milk and honey. Canaan was the Promised Land. What land has He promised to bring you to? Are you willing to let go of the past to be transitioned into something new?

God gave Moses instructions for entering the Promise Land: "*Send men to scout out the country of Canaan that I am giving to the people of Israel. Send one man from each tribe.*" Moses obediently sent out a spy from each of the twelve tribes of Israel. The spies departed from the Valley of

Eschol and spied the land for forty days; they brought back one cluster of grapes and some of the pomegranates and figs, showing that the land was fruitful. Their report: "... *We went to the land where you sent us. It truly flows with milk and honey, and this is its fruit. Nevertheless the people who dwell in the land are strong, the cities are fortified and very large, moreover we saw the descendents of Anak there*" (Numbers 13:27, 28 NKJV) The Anaks were a race of giants, descendants of the Anakim who lived in Canaan, the Promised Land. For the Israelites the giants probably brought back memories of enslavement while in Egypt; fear crept in, immobilized, and paralyzed them from reaching their purpose.

The Hebrew word *Nephilim,* from *nephil*, means "giant," "tyrant," or "bully." The term refers to a tall race of people, men of great stature. The Israelites were not supposed to look at the people of the land but were to trust God in His ability to protect them as He protected them from Pharaoh and the Egyptian army. However, God's people began to see themselves through their own eyes and forgot the promises of God. God had given the land to the Israelites to possess through the covenant agreement made with Abraham, Isaac, Jacob, and Moses. God's covenant was an everlasting promise to Abraham before his son Isaac was born; and God never changed His mind about Abraham's inheritance.

> *And I will establish my covenant between Me and you and your descendants after you in their generations, for an everlasting covenant, to be God to you and your descendants after you. "Also I give to you and your descendants after you the land in which you are a stranger, all the land of Canaan, as an everlasting possession; and I will be their God ....* (Genesis 17:7, 8 NKJV).

The ten spies who were intimidated by the stature of the residents of the land needed deliverance from an old mindset; for while in Egypt, they had been devalued and as a result developed low self esteem as slaves. So fearful of the inhabitants of the land, the ten spies cried out and declared:

> *We are not able to go up against the people, for they are stronger than we... The land through which we have gone as spies is a land that devours its inhabitants, and all the peopl whom we saw in it are men of great stature. There we saw the giants (the descendants of Anak came from the giants); and we were like grasshoppers in our own sight, and so we were in their sight* (Numbers 13:31, 32b, 33 NKJV).

The ten Israelite spies' low self-worth affected their ability to recognize their potential; they believed it was useless to try and take the Promised Land. The ten spies saw themselves as failures, and therefore unable to take Canaan according to God's promise. They needed inner healing from such disabling and devaluing thoughts. They, unlike Caleb, failed to speak life. They would have benefited from agreeing with Caleb and Joshua, who believed that the Israelites could possess the land. Spiritually, the other spies were not prepared: "*Death and life are in the power of the tongue and those who love it will eat its fruit*" (Proverbs 18:21 NKJV).

As slaves they were not allowed to possess, subdue, or have dominion over anything. Even though they had been in the presence of God and had been given a champion as a leader, they had not matured on their spiritual journey. The leaders of their tribes were fragile, fearful, faultfinding, faulty, and foolish. Indeed they had left Egypt, where they had been enslaved for over 400 years, but they were never liberated from the slave mentality. They also had a spirit of worldliness on them—*Egypt* being synonymous with *worldliness.*

It took Moses 40 years to be liberated from the culture of Egypt in order to prepare for one of the most supernatural deliverances in the history of biblical text. It took him another 40 years to get to know the ways of God, after having been reared as an Egyptian, in order for him to have complete confidence in God to accomplish the task, to be victorious.

While sitting in the New Birth Cathedral, I have heard Bishop Eddie L. Long, Senior Pastor of New Birth Missionary Baptist in Lithonia, Georgia, say numerous times, "Your down time is your preparation time." It is time that should be spent in preparation through studying the Word of God, in prayer, and in fellowship with Him.

The Israelites did not understand that they could overthrow their enemies with God's help and possess the land; they needed inner healing from old memories and deliverance from the spirit of fear. When they saw the giants, it probably reminded them of their past as bond-servants held in captivity against their will; and they immediately became fearful due to their physical size. Fear will immobilize, paralyze, and demoralize an individual or a group of people; it is a stronghold sent from Satan's kingdom. Fear also carries with it torment. Fear is a spirit and is transferable. The ten went back to their camp in fear because it brought back memories of the past, and caused the entire congregation to be in torment or agony.

After the congregation heard the report of the ten spies, they lifted up their voices and cried, and the people wept all night.

> *All the Israelites grumbled against Moses and Aaron, and the whole assembly said to them, "If only we had died in Egypt! Or in this desert! Why is the LORD bringing us to this land only to let us fall by the sword? Our wives and children will be taken as plunder. Wouldn't it be better for us to go back to Egypt?* (Numbers 14:2, 3 NIV).

The spies' negative report caused the people great despair. The culture they were accustomed to had been birthed in a negative environment. Today, as then, you may hear some individuals claim when believing their trials to be so cumbersome, "I almost lost my mind." This may have been what some of the Hebrew children were experiencing as they thought about and focused on their past lifestyle. Some people cannot advance beyond their past experiences.

They were disturbed and this caused them to forget the miracles that God had done for them. They failed to realize that God is without any character flaws, that He has to uphold His reputation; for He cannot lie. "*God is not a man, that he should lie; neither the son of man, that he should repent: hath he said, and shall he not do it? Or hath he spoken, and shall he not make it good*?" (Numbers 23:19) Fear will change your perspective on life. The apostle Paul taught the young pastor Timothy about this spirit, saying, "*For God has not given us a spirit of fear, but of power and of love and of a sound mind*" (2 Timothy 1:7 NKJV). It is so important not to become intimidated because intimidation minimizes effectiveness.

Fear is a stronghold that keeps people in bondage: Some fear losing their income, some fear their children will be harmed or injured, and others fear the ramifications of new healthcare laws. During this term of President Barak Obama, many individuals fear changes that are being made by our President and the legislators. Fear is a spirit which comes to antagonize, assault, worry, horrify, agitate, disable, and to make a person lose their sense of identity as a believer. "*Fear not, for I am with you; Be not dismayed, for I am your God. I will strengthen you, Yes, I will help you, I will uphold you with My righteous right hand*" (Isaiah 41:10 NKJV).

Fear is the opposite of faith. Dr. Myles Monroe states in *Releasing Your Potential: Exposing the Hidden You:* "Faith requires you to function by believing first, instead of seeing or feeling first. Living by faith also requires that you put your soul under the control of your spirit. Your soul governs your emotions, will, and mind. When you live from your soul, you allow information from your physical body to govern your decisions. Your soul may say, "I'm unhappy because the outward circumstance of my life is not what I would like for it to be." Just because you don't feel what God is saying to you, don't refuse to believe that He does not know what He is talking about. We have to trust in Him, wait on Him, and rely on His Word when we cannot see our way."

One Hebrew word for fear is *pachad,* which means alarm: dread . . . great fear . . . terror. Such fear causes you to be frightened, to be made afraid or to feel dreadful. Israel had an unnecessary and unhealthy fear of the nations of Canaan. People can be in the midst of where God is doing awesome things and still miss Him. I have heard some believers declare, "I will not miss the day of my visitation." We must not miss God when He is trying to transition us into something new either.

Joshua and Caleb admonished the people concerning God's will for them: "*Only do not rebel against the LORD. And do not be afraid of the people of the land, because we will swallow them up. Their protection is gone, but the LORD is with us. Do not be afraid of them*" (Numbers 14: 9 NIV). The Israelites were relying on their souls and, therefore, were not able to reach their potential. After reading their story, it is tragic to realize that some individuals never came into the blessings God had for them. There were others who had to suffer because of the rebellious and stubborn spirit of the majority. Individuals need to see themselves made in the image and likeness of God in order to avoid low self esteem or self devaluation. Because fear paralyzes, demoralizes, or discourages, it can be instrumental in hindering God's plan for your life.

God has given Christian believers the power to bind the spirit of fear and command it to come out, to let go of an individual. It is a spirit, and it can come and go. Once again: *"For God hath not given us the spirit of fear; but of power, and of love, and of a sound mind"* (2 Timothy 1:7). The fear that brings dread or apprehension is also the source of phobias that exist in the world. I John 4:18 states, "*There is no fear in love; but perfect love casteth out fear: because fear hath torment. He that feareth is not made perfect in love.*" We have been encouraged not to fear according to the Word of God. When you hear a negative report, fear may come in; however, you can cast down fear by using the Word of God. I am talking about fear that dominates and controls your life through imaginations and thoughts. We have to cast down negative thoughts and imaginations. "*Casting down imaginations, and every high thing that exalteth itself against the knowledge of God, and bringing into captivity every thought to the obedience of Christ*" (2 Corinthians 10: 5).

The spirit of fear will allow an individual or groups of individuals to devalue their worth and keep their mind in captivity in order to prevent their progress. This was the case with the Israelites. Initially the spirit of fear attacks your mind, which is within your soul, along with your emotions and your will. Wage war against this spirit when you see it plotting to overtake you. Emotional fear may occur when you suffer a near accident but it is short lived and different from fear that brings torment. Fear that dominates, controls, and discredits is from the demonic realm; rebuke it, and take authority over it.

Rebuke (it means to order with authority) and bind up the spirit of fear; decree and declare it is rendered powerless and ineffective against you. Declare that you loose power, love, and a sound mind over your thoughts and imaginations. Jesus has given you the power to bind and loose . . . He has given us these keys of authority as a church: "*Assuredly, I say to you, whatever you bind on earth will be bound in heaven, and whatever you loose on earth will be loosed in heaven*" (Matthew 18:18 NKJV). Avoid seeing yourself through the eyes of others and see yourself through the eyes of God. Believe, "*I can do all things through Christ who strengthens me*" (Philippians 4:13 NKJV).

4

BE SET FREE: INNER HEALING

Flora Slosson Wuellner authored *Release: Healing from Wounds of Family, Church, and Community* in which she focuses on environmental, climatic, generational and soul-tie issues as being responsible for our negative conditions. She states, "The dark wounding through the generations, the toxicity in communities around us, has begun to enter our consciousness in many ways. We see the ancient, inherited shadows between the warring nations and the bitterly embattled great ethnic groups. We see the generational burdens in our families, and the wounds we absorb from one another, the energy drained in our personal relationships."

Wuellner goes on to ask, "Is the pain of our communal bodies the new frontier of healing? Can this vast pain that spans decades, even centuries, be healed? Can we personally be healed by God and set free from the burden and the bleeding? How can one pray for inherited and absorbed wounding? Far more than we realize, we inherit emotional burdens, communal darkness, experience heavy draining like a chronic emotional hemorrhaging from our relationships, and the groups to which we belong." This reflects the burden and bleeding of others who are present in the same environment with us and are infected with wounds, sufferings, pains, and maladies that are caught by association, and through our environment.

Inner healing is necessary in order to be set free from stuff and junk that have wounded many individuals without them being aware of it. Even ministers, pastors, counselors, and lay leaders experience the toxicity of their surroundings. The word *inner* has various meanings such as: inside, inward, internal, intimate, central, deep rooted, inherit, etc. Proverbs 18:14 states in the New Revised Standard Version, "*The spirit of a person will sustain their infirmity, but a wounded spirit who can bear it?*" The human spirit or soul represents the seat of emotions, the mind, and the will. God breathed on humankind and we became a living soul. The word "soul" is a feminine noun describing both the inner being with its thoughts and emotions. The person who needs inner healing must have the emotional, spiritual, and the interpersonal aspects of their lives examined; this being necessary in order to ascertain the root of the problem for complete deliverance.

Flora Slosson Wuellner further discusses how association with others can influence an individual. She believes that we take risks and are vulnerable, that is, when we choose to love people. She asserts that this is "empowered vulnerability," which means "the love that has been set free by God to choose freely, to take risks, to reach out, to withdraw, to suffer, to give from a deep center that has been released from prisons of all kinds. . . . When we are moved by love to reach out and rescue another person who is drowning in emotional crises and anguish, it is a love that does not disempower either the rescuer or the rescued." We do not have to be fearful of assisting someone in their deliverance from bondage of any sort; just be prepared.

Love, for some, represents being in bondage to a degree . . . not so for Jesus who was never in bondage while demonstrating love. He was able to separate Himself from the conditions around Him. He did not absorb the evil around Him but confronted evil and spoke truth to powers. In the midst of Jesus' preaching, teaching, healing, and restoring He had to address emotional, ethnic, generational, and environmental issues to liberate others. There were some who doubted; others who tried to dispose of Him; and a few who were so religious and traditional, they refused to receive His ministry of liberation.

At the time of this writing, I am a wife, mother, pastor, teacher, intercessor, counselor, and nurse. I am an "apostolic mother"—having been engaged in the ministry of deliverance, healing, and restoration for over twenty years. Our ministry has been effective in liberating individuals from various forms of bondages; however, some individuals were not liberated. I have come to find out that an individual has to desire to be set free . . . otherwise trying to take someone through the process will be futile. There have been some who came through the ministry but refused to admit that they needed help. Sadly, you must pray for them and ask God to continue sending someone their way that they can learn to trust enough to receive their breakthrough. Sometimes they are not ready to let go of their past . . . sometimes their past may be too painful for them to allow it to surface. Suppression of painful memories is a way of coping for some individuals. Help may be available; nevertheless, it has to be their decision.

God has many ways to help those who are hurting. He uses the five-fold ministry gifts— the apostle, prophet, evangelist, pastor and teacher—to be a blessing in edifying and equipping others. God also gives believers the spiritual gifts which allow us to operate through the power of the Holy Spirit, for the profit of all. The process of deliverance may begin by God speaking, from the mouth of a man or woman of God, concerning your past or your present state. (This is one of the gifts of the Spirit recorded in 1 Corinthians 12:8.) When a *word of knowledge* is spoken in the presence of a person who is in bondage, he or she has to know this is God using the one speaking.

The process of deliverance begins many times from the point of the individual receiving the revelation, even to the point of the person beginning to cry because what is being revealed is truth. After their past or present state has been revealed, the individual is encouraged or exhorted to make a decision about the direction to take. If they are ready to be free, the Holy Spirit will open the eyes of their understanding to what is available. What seemed hopeless before is suddenly possible, because now they can see the light. "*God is our refuge and strength, a very present help in trouble*" (Psalm 46:1).

Flora Slosson Wuellner shares, there were some women who worked with me and, after a period of time, I was able to discern that they were influencing me by their association. The things they were spewing out of their mouths were, at times, done in a subtle way but were very infectious. The air in the room became congested with an emotional virus. A virus is a microorganism that spreads by air droplets, bodily fluids, or objects. It can be identified by a microscope, and it is responsible for sickness, diseases, and various illnesses. Working with these people became very draining: I became very tired and could not explain my tiredness. A close friend warned that I was being drained by sources that were around me. An emotional virus is like a python spirit that comes to squeeze the life out of you. It becomes necessary for your well being to remove yourself from the environment or limit your association with it.

When I was married previously, neither my spouse nor I was committed to living a Christian life. I attended church, yet my heart was far from having a relationship with God. Due to my husband's jealousy, domestic violence often occurred—usually initiated by his alcohol use. Dishonesty was prevalent in our relationship. Later it was adultery, bar hopping, and his refusal to pay child support that led to a permanent separation, and finally divorce. After a season of being in that environment, it became easy for me to engage in fighting back in self defense, engaging in foul language, and dating other men—wanting "to get even." The foul things that came out of my ex-husband's mouth soon infected me and I found myself using profanity as often as he did. It became an issue when my youngest son began repeating the curse words that came out of my mouth. My incontinence, in the use of certain words, had affected my youngest child; and I am sure it affected the oldest two children, but, fortunately, they were of an age not to repeat what was heard.

Emotionally, I was hurt from the marital relationship: Every time I would ask him to leave or forcibly put him out, he would later return. Domestic violence was really a big issue even during the honeymoon stage, but it always seemed as if things were going to improve. It did not. Ours was a continuous cycle of separation due to the repeated violence and dysfunction. It was impossible for our relationship to work because we both needed a relationship with the Lord Jesus. He needed deliverance from alcohol, drugs, anger, and being physically-emotionally abusive. I needed deliverance from a competitive spirit; from provoking my spouse at times; from low self esteem, insecurity, a foul mouth, anger, and unforgiveness. I felt pain, shame, regret, anger, and at the same held a little faith in the improvement of our relationship. It was false hope! Things will never improve in a relationship unless at least one person submits to Christ wholeheartedly:

> *For the unbelieving husband is sanctified by the wife, and the unbelieving wife is sanctified by the husband; else were your children unclean, but now are they holy? But if the unbelieving depart, let him depart. A brother or a sister is not under bondage in such cases; but God hath called us to peace* (1 Corinthians 7:14, 15).

Neither of us had someone to speak positively into our situation or a counselor to assist us in our relationship. Pastoral counseling would have been great, but I was in fellowship with a church that was "secular" in its approach. I was too ashamed to discuss my situation with a pastor because I did not want to disclose personal information. I was filled with so much anger at times that I wanted to kill my finance. And at one time in our relationship, I nearly did . . . shot him with a twenty-two caliber gun aimed at his head; but he shut the door and the bullet hit him in his arm! He did not press charges. Now that should have been enough for me to separate from him, and I did—but I always allowed him to return. Clearly, you must see why it is not worth being in an abusive relationship because lives are sometimes lost. In that life you cheat yourself from reaching your potential.

My father was abusive to my mother. After leaving the Navy at twenty-one years of age, Dad married Mother and together they had four children—one child every year for four years. Some might say that we were "stair steps." My paternal grandmother spoke of my dad being "shell shocked" while in the Navy; that it affected him mentally, which was obvious only when he drank alcohol. He resorted to a life of alcohol abuse, becoming very abusive to my mother. We could not live together as a family because of his alcoholism, physical abuse, anger, mentally revisiting World War Two episodes, and refusal to commit to his marriage vows. Due to my parents' unique situation, my paternal grandmother reared their children.

It is wise to receive marriage counseling before getting married. Sometimes previous relationships can hurt a new relationship if both parties are not completely honest with each other; and I am sure my mother and dad both had issues that contributed to their marital problems. It is necessary to find out some history about your future mate and his or her family to avoid surprises later on in the relationship. Once again, my parents were not actively involved in church at the time we were born, nor did my dad have a relationship with Christ. I have come to a place in my Christian walk to understand that many issues could have been avoided if their lives had been centered on Jesus Christ. Today, my mother is a born-again Christian and she loves the Lord! She is such a meek, humble, quiet, and loving person, loved by all who meet her.

Issues of life can flow into an individual's life and sabotage their destiny. Each offspring must make a conscious decision not to stay in the same rut as their parents, or stay in bad situations they have gotten involved in. I had to walk away from a bad marriage and charge ahead toward a new lifestyle; and it was not easy. I went into the next relationship with "issues" because I had not been delivered from those things that previously held me captive. The new relationship was less dramatic, therefore allowing me space to rediscover who I was and to renew my relationship with God. In my brokenness I was able to discover a caring God—not immediately, but at my own pace. One day while visiting a local church, I had an encounter that began for me a life-changing process. This gives pause to examine the biblical woman with the issue of blood and the challenges she faced.

Consider that this woman's "issue of blood" is one that caused females to be separated from others—her running issue subjected her to other issues. The Luke narrative (story) speaks of this woman's suffering from pain, shame, and agony—a woman who was seemingly hopeless until she decided to do something ridiculous:

> *Now a woman having, a flow of blood for twelve years, who had spent all her livelihood on physicians and could not be healed by any, came from behind and touched the border of His garment. And immediately her flow of blood stopped. And Jesus said, "Who touched me?" When all denied it, Peter and those with him said, "Master, the multitudes throng and press You, and You say, 'Who touched Me?'" But Jesus said, "Somebody touched Me, for I perceived power going out from Me." Now when the woman saw that she was not hidden, she came trembling; and falling down before Him, she declared to Him in the presence of all the people the reason she had touched Him and how she was healed immediately. And He said to her, "Daughter, be of good cheer; your faith has made you well. Go in peace (Luke 8:43-48 NKJV).*

It took fortitude for this woman to touch a rabbi and to declare her healing without seeing a priest. This is the kind of faith the Lord is looking for throughout the earth; faith that commands some corresponding action for whatever you believe God for.

The woman with the issue of blood was a person who represents those needing inner healing as well as bodily healing. This woman was in crisis—brought on by the longevity of her illness, the financial strain, emotional pain, and the loss of blood that supplied oxygen to all cells. She needed holistic healing. In other words she needed her total person set free, for she experienced great shame and pain. Dr. Edward P. Wimberly in his work, *Moving from Shame to Self-Worth,* identifies sufferers of shame as "people who believe they are flawed and unlovable. They need time in caring relationships before they are able to respond to any idea that God might care for them." He further states, "Devastating shame blocks people's ability to discern a caring God."

Matthew 9:20, 22 (NIV) also discloses Jesus' encounter with the woman with an issue of blood (same narrative told by two different historians):

> *Just then a woman who had been subject to bleeding for twelve years came up behind Him and touched His cloak. She said to herself, 'If only I may touch His cloak, I will be healed.' "Jesus turned and saw her, 'Take heart, daughter,' He said; 'Your faith has healed you.' And the woman was healed from that moment.*

For twelve years the woman with the issue of blood had expected a cure from different physicians, but it did not happen. Can you imagine the shame, humiliation, hurt, and disappointment she must have felt? She must have been broken on the inside due to the repeatedly negative reports from the physicians. Have you ever been in a situation like this? This woman became deliberate in her desperation to receive healing—desperation that finally moved her to seek healing from the Lord. In doing so she even found herself going against the Jewish Law; but so serious was she about receiving deliverance that it resulted in a radical move of faith: She believed…acted on her belief… and obtained favorable results. The Book of James reveals to us that there must be some action to correspond with our faith: "*. . . faith by itself, if it is not accompanied by action, is dead*" (James 2:17 NIV).

> *As the Scripture says, "Anyone who trusts in Him will never be put to shame. Not all the Israelites accepted the good news. For Isaiah says, "Lord, who Has believed our message?" Consequently, faith comes from hearing the message, and the message [the Gospel] is heard through the word of Christ* (Romans 10:11, 16, 17 NIV).

I continue to expound on the woman with the issue of blood because of her supernatural faith that was made known in an uncommon situation. News has a way of getting around fast whether it is positive or negative. Even though this woman with the issue of blood was not to be seen mingling with the public, the news about Jesus, the Healer, reached her ears. "*So then faith comes by hearing, and hearing by the word of God*" (Romans 10:17 NKJV). It is so important for an individual to believe in the promises of God; for you can always put God in remembrance of His Word. Our actions should always correspond with our faith or belief when we hear news that can turn our situation around.

This woman knew the *Torah* (first five books of the Hebrew Bible) and the promises of God, which included healing. God made a healing covenant with the Israelites while they were in the wilderness. God spoke to Moses their leader who obediently informed the people:

> *If you diligently heed the voice of the Lord your God and do what is right in His sight, give ear to His commandments and keep all His statutes, I will put none of the diseases on you which I have brought on the Egyptians; for I am LORD who heals you* (Exodus 15:26 NKJV).

Following the laws of God in the *Torah* was designed to keep individuals free from sickness and various diseases. Not appropriating the Laws would result in curses coming upon the Israelites. God established a covenant with His people if they would follow and obey Him He would protect them. If they refused to obey it would expose them to unusual circumstances with unfavorable results by their own decision.

Sexual immorality leads to sexually transmitted diseases, such as: AIDS, Chlamydia, Gonorrhea and others. God's Law is purposeful to keep you sound in spirit, soul, and body; it is the application of the Word of God that keeps individuals in spiritual, physical, mental, and emotional health, as well as economic stability. There are other systems that affect uniformity of humanity, such as, the political and social justice system, but God is our defense—He has the Master Plan. Disruption in these systems may cause you to be unbalanced or to experience a lack of equilibrium in your total person; but this does not have to be! We are told by our Creator to pray and not to worry, but meditate upon God's Word, and speak the Word over yourselves and your situations.

The woman with the issue of blood was not worried about the threatening possibility of religious leaders stoning her for touching a rabbi. She needed to be made whole; her life was not fruitful, and she desperately desired change. In frustration she made a last attempt to survive; and worrying about what others thought was not an issue at that time. Worry is a symptom of the spirit of fear; it is a symptom of an inner problem, especially when it consumes your thoughts and incapacitates you. When an individual is worried to the point of giving up, faith cannot be exercised to receive the promises of God.

Looking at things in the natural will at times discourage you; yet we serve a supernatural God who is doing supernatural things for his sons and daughters. It is time to be radically bold, to be deliberate in our intentions, and to aim at our targets for definite recovery. There are adversaries who are deceptive and cunning. We have to know our position as Kingdom of God people, and we have to set our faces like a flint, determined not to move. This woman was bold and deliberate; she knew what her purpose was, and so touched the hem of Jesus' garment as she had settled [that issue] in her heart. I keep emphasizing the story about this woman because it is the radical exercise of her faith that I want you to understand that caused her to receive deliverance and holistic well-being. She was set free spirit, soul (mind, emotions, and will), and body.

Sometimes answers to prayers are not received because of wavering faith. This woman had no time to waiver; she was determined to only touch Jesus' hem; it is important to be specific about your intentions. She had the wisdom to know it was not time to play games; this may have been her only and last opportunity to be healed; so it was critical to move as God was leading her. This woman was determined not to miss her day of visitation! I believe there was an appointment set up for her to get through the crowd to touch Jesus. At her set time—"*kairos*" moment—or predetermined time, no one could hinder her. There are established times God has for you to receive, as well as for you to perform certain things, and you will not be hindered during your season. This is not your season to fail if you can [believe and] receive it!

James emphasizes how to receive wisdom and the importance of petitioning God in faith:

> *If any of you lacks wisdom, let him ask of God, who gives to all liberally and without reproach, and it will be given to him. But let him ask in faith, with no doubting, for he who doubts is like a wave of the sea driven and tossed by the wind. For let not that man suppose that he will receive anything from the Lord; he is a double-minded man, unstable in all his ways* (James 1:5-8 NKJV).

He says here that the one who possesses wisdom also possesses knowledge with ability to make wise decisions in adverse conditions. Wisdom is knowledge guided by understanding.

The woman with the issue of blood knew in her heart when to press in to receive her miracle. It was a miracle because her twelve-year flow of blood ceased immediately. She had made up her mind that she was not going to leave Jesus' presence until He blessed her. What a demonstration of faith in God! What do you believe God for? Keep on declaring and decreeing it as you ask the Father in Jesus name.

What is your issue? Is it drugs, alcohol, food addiction, sexual perversion, such as: pornography, identity crises in your sexuality, a child pervert or are you involved in some other form of sexual misconduct such as adultery or fornication? Is it sickness, disease, or some other kind of infirmity? Or are you engaged in witchcraft, horoscope reading, or maybe it is speaking doubt and unbelief? You can be delivered by confessing your faults to the Lord. Ask the Lord to set you free. Denounce your sins; ask Him to forgive you. Ask Him once again to set you free, unapologetically. Quit asking in fear as if Jesus is unapproachable; ask in full assurance that He hears, that He cares, and that He will deliver you. He is very approachable to you even in all of your mess. I know because he was approachable to me in all of my mess, and He is still working on my character so that it will be a reflection of His character. I have not arrived at perfection yet.

I want to encourage you . . . I know this to be true because He has been there for me even when I did not realize it. Through the power of the Holy Spirit, you will be released from bondage when you sincerely petition God's help. Salvation is for all people who will call upon the name of Jesus. Only you and God know what you are really dealing with. Everyone has some desires that they cannot share with others, but I say to you be transparent, ask for help, from the right source.

The apostle Peter was sent to preach the gospel to a man (Cornelius) and his family who were not Jews, and thus discerned from the Holy Spirit: "*And Peter opened his mouth and said: Most certainly and thoroughly I now perceive and understand that God shows no partiality and is no respecter of persons*" (Acts 10:34 AMP). Jesus had set the example for Peter and for all believers:

Jesus went throughout Galilee, teaching in the synagogues, preaching the good news of the kingdom, and healing every disease and sickness among the people. News about Him spread all over Syria, and people brought to Him all who were ill with various diseases, those suffering severe pain, the demonized, those having seizures, and the paralyzed, and he healed them (Matthew 4:23, 24 NIV).

Jesus took our punishment so that humanity could be healed and saved. There are "thirty seven diseases and infirmities" named in the Bible. "These and many other unidentified sicknesses and infirmities have been healed by God, as recorded in both testaments. Full provision has been made by Christ to heal all physical ailments" (Dake's). *"That it might be fulfilled which was spoken by Isaiah the prophet, saying, Himself took our infirmities, and bare our sicknesses,"* Matthew 8:17. The ultimate redemption by atonement is not only to remove all sin, but also all sickness with complete redemption of body as well as soul" (Dake's, page 8).

Jesus was taken before Pontius Pilate, the Roman governor, who made the final decision about His crucifixion. Pilate was hesitant to give the religious leaders permission to crucify Jesus initially; but they threatened to report him to the Roman emperor, Caesar; and Pilate could not afford to have his job in jeopardy. He was hired to keep the peace but now a tumult was rising among the Jewish people; they demanded Barabbas' release and Jesus' crucifixion. "*Then he released Barabbas to them; and when he had scourged [beaten, flogged] Jesus, he delivered Him to be crucified*" (Matthew 27:26 NKJV).

According to Dake's "A scourge was a Roman implement for severe bodily punishment. It consisted of a handle with about a dozen leather cords with jagged pieces of bone or metal at each end to make the blow more painful and effective . . . . Flogging was permitted by law up to forty stripes. Jews reduced this to thirty-nine stripes. If the scourge used on Jesus had twelve thongs and he was hit even thirty-nine times, this would make 468 stripes."

The cross is often referenced, and rightfully so, concerning the removal of sins through the shed blood of Christ, while the other part of the cross experience is often left out or either touched upon lightly. Jesus bore our sins, sicknesses and diseases. Once you see all sickness, disease, and infirmities on Him, you will no longer claim them as yours. The woman with the issue of blood took the risk to get to Jesus because she had heard the reports that others were being made whole. She recognized her inner, personal issues that needed to be resolved. She went to Jesus knowing that her shame, low self-esteem, loneliness and fear would be vanquished. She went to Jesus knowing that she would find the love, acceptance, and complete healing she desired.

The Book of Leviticus is a book of laws established for the people as a pattern of life. God gave the Israelite community guidelines to help them to be organized as a people with high values reflecting God's holiness. As such consider Leviticus 15:25-27 (NKJV):

> *If a woman has a discharge of blood for many days, other than at the time of her customary impurity, or if it runs beyond her usual time of impurity, all the days of her unclean discharge shall be as the days of her customary impurity. She shall be unclean. Every bed on which she lies all the days of her discharge*

> *shall be to her as the bed of impurity; and whatever she sits on shall be unclean, as the uncleanness of her impurity. Whoever touches those things shall be unclean; he shall wash his clothes and bathe in water, and be unclean until evening.*

What was so great about touching Jesus' garment? Was there power in the garment? Is there power in the garments of those who represent Christ? The Greek word for "garment" is *himatiŏn*, which denotes a "dress—inner or outer, raiment, clothes, cloak, robe, vesture, apparel." It is, in other words, an outer cloak or mantle thrown over the *chiton*, the Greek word for an "undergarment" usually worn next to the skin, a garment, a vestment. This is important because these garments represented a legal process at one time according to Matthew 5:40: When going before a court of law, the claimant was suppose to claim the less costly garment—the inner vest. When the Roman soldiers seized Jesus, they took His garments—the inner and outer apparels.

After she touched Jesus, the virtue, the power, and the anointing went out of Him, and the woman was declared whole. The Greek word for "whole" is *sōzō*, which means to save, deliver, protect, make whole, heal, or do well. She was delivered from sickness and suffering by exercising her faith in Christ the Healer. Her shame left her and there was no need for her to feel inferior. The woman was timid, slow to acknowledge her deliverance at first; but fear immediately subsided, because the thing she probably feared the most had been done—she had touched a rabbi and had not been stoned to death. Her action was done secretly; however, Jesus exposed the realm of faith in which she operated at that time to the masses.

The moment she was recognized by Jesus her self-worth increased and loneliness vanished like a flick of lightning. Being in the presence of God changes your atmosphere; so that you are able to recover from the everyday challenges that life brings. The very aroma of healing prayers set the tone for your deliverance from inner pain and shame. As believers we have to take authority over the atmosphere through prayer and bind up influences that may be infectious.

A wounded person may walk in constant strife because of possessing feelings of rejection, insecurity, or inadequacy Such a person needs inner healing—that is, spiritual and emotional healing. Repeated insults of rejection can altar one's ability to trust; thereby, resulting in a suspicion of others. God wants the person to trust in Him; for inner healing comes through developing a loving, lasting relationship with God. As a result of developing a relationship of trust with God, other meaningful relationships can be formed and kept. Toxicity in your surroundings has to be identified to be separated from the source. Who is influencing you that would have a negative impact on life? Are you surrounding yourself with people who are dream killers? Who is speaking into your purpose to help propel you into the direction that has been destined for you to take before the foundation of the earth? Who are you associating with that believes life is meaningless or it is worthless to envision doing great things?

Emotional, relational and communal influences are relevant in inner sufferings. These influences can occur in your church, your family, and your work place—just a few places for you to examine why you are being invaded by something that did not originate within you. Flora Slosson Wuellner's observation is valid: You can be influenced by your associations; your environment; your influences, as well as family genetics or DNA.

We live in a community with people who have many issues; and it is often not one person's fault. It is almost impossible to live in an environment that does not make a person conducive to these prerequisites. One example would be a child who was molested by a relative, or by a stranger. Did that child do anything to deserve this kind of treatment? No!—It was madness or a demonic force in the individual who performed the horrendous act. Did it originate within the child? No, but it will more than likely affect the child to withdraw from loving relationships, or to possibly imitate the sexual act that was performed on them later on in life.

There are various types of environmental toxins we need to be aware of that infect and inflict the natural body and, ultimately, involve the inner aspects of an individual soul. Allow me to offer the following example: Some folk contracted the *Swine Flu*, a virus that had the ability to make one terminally ill, until the vaccine was given. Not only did it affect one's body, it also affected the thought processes. When a person faces an illness, many times such thoughts flood their mind as: *Am I going to get better? Will I live? Will I be permanently disabled and have to depend on others to assist me in life's daily activities?* Illness affects your emotions, evidenced at times by periods of crying, of anxiety, fear, prolonged grief, inadequacies, inferiority, or other emotional issues. There are times when some folk may give up or lose their will to fight after a bout of sickness. This is the reason why each individual needs to keep their spirit edified or built up in the Word of God. When illness or any unforeseen events happen, you can rely on your inner strength to help you gain the momentum to fight. It is important to learn how to fight the good fight of faith; even if you are unable to speak the Word aloud, your inner spirit speaks to your heart and thoughts, emotions and will—encouraging you to not give up. Therefore when someone visits you and speaks the

Word of God over you, it agrees with your spirit. Even when your intellect tries to remind you of the report your physician has given you or your family while standing over your bed, you have the strength to reject and renounce it. Faith is now operating!

Somewhere in your mind you remember the old song sung by your mother, or grandmother, or a church deacon. Maybe your spirit begins humming "I Will Trust in the Lord Until I Die." We know that we are translated from this life to a new life in Christ. It may also be that you are not able to readily sing at this point in your illness but you feel a choir on the inside of your belly; so singing the "Songs of Zion" will encourage your spirit to live and declare the works of the Lord. We have been given the power to declare and decree a thing in Jesus' name—and it shall come to pass.

Remember, what you say is what you get. *"Therefore I say to you, whatsoever things you ask when you pray, believe that you receive them, and you will have them*" (Mark 11:24). You may need to keep confessing it until it manifests; so therefore, continue in faith, with the assurance that God hears . . . He cares and He will answer. Do not allow outward circumstances to change your confession; speak those things that are not as though they were. God is never too early, nor too late—God is always on time! There is a set time that He has decided for you to receive your blessings. Another song I recall hearing often in my childhood testifies to the same truth: "You Can't Hurry God." Yes, God operates in His own timing; but if you wait on the Lord, He will renew your strength and He will fulfill His promises to you. Thus, the question the Old Testament prophet Isaiah asks of believers:

> *Have you not known? Have you not heard? The everlasting God, the LORD, the Creator of the ends of the*

earth, neither faints nor is weary. His understanding is unsearchable. He gives power to the weak, And to those who have no might He increases strength. Even the youths shall faint and be weary, and the young men shall utterly fall, But those who wait on the LORD, shall renew their strength; they shall mount up with wings like eagles; they shall run and not be weary, they shall walk and not faint" (Isaiah 40:28-31 NKJV).

In spite of our human weaknesses and frailties, our source of power is God. As long as we wait in expectancy and in confidence and in assurance, our due season is coming. We must allow ourselves to be spiritually renewed while waiting; waiting in prayer, in meditation, in confessing the Word of God, in praise and worship, and in giving. It is a Kingdom of God principle that when we give, God gives back to us immeasurable amounts. Keep sowing and cultivating your seed until due harvest time arrives. When our due season comes, we will mount up and soar like an eagle. The Hebrew-Greek Bible explains that "the Hebrew word for mount up is *kawvaw,* a verb meaning to bind together, collect, to expect, gather together, look, tarry, and wait; to wait for, to look for, and to hope for. The word is used to signify depending on and ordering activities around a future event."

Be set free; allow yourself to see the need for God to be present in your deliverance and healing. It is time for the brokenhearted to be healed by the power of God; and it does not have to be a process . . . but it is according to your mindset, belief, or the seed sown into you. Jesus delivered individuals the moment they came into His presence. Once we have an encounter with the Lord Jesus, we can no longer remain the same; so be set free!

When we pray for healing and it does not seem to be effective, it is because we carry the desolations of many generations. There are generational curses that must be broken, because these will try to defeat you and your blood line. God told the Israelites that He was "*. . . a jealous God visiting the iniquity (wickedness) of the fathers upon the children unto the third and fourth generations of those who hate Me*" (Exodus 20:5 NKJV). The Lord gave me this verse fourteen years ago: "*And they shall build the old wastes, they shall raise up the former desolations, and they shall repair the waste cities, the desolations of many generations*" (Isaiah 61:4).

Believers have been given authority to trample on Satan and his kingdom of darkness: "*Behold, I give unto you power to tread on serpents and scorpions, and over all the power of the enemy, and nothing shall by any means hurt you*" (Luke 10:19). We have been given power through repentance, prayer, and renunciation to break and destroy generational curses; from incest to abortions, including addictions such as alcohol, prescription drugs and street drugs; from sexual immorality, including pornography, gender aberration; from divorce, domestic violence, and many others adverse behaviors.

When the redemptive work of Calvary is accepted as a resolution to any addiction or sexual perversion, we will witness mighty deliverances. The blood of Jesus was shed for the forgiveness of our sins. Jesus appeared to His disciples several times within the forty days after His Resurrection and reminded them, and us: "*Whosoever sins you remit [forgive], they are remitted [forgiven] unto them, and whosoever sins you retain, they are retained*" (John 20:23).

5

INNER HEALING FOR WOUNDS SUPERFICIALLY CURED

Many physical maladies would not exist if inner healing had already occurred in an individual. Many sicknesses stem from inner pain and suffering that could be alleviated with the right coach or mentor to assist individuals through to their deliverance. The problem is that some coaches or mentors do not deal with the internal issues on a spiritual level for the person suffering. In her book *Release,* Flora Wuellner Slosson addresses the issue of not being "prepared in prayer" to assist in bringing inner healing to those in need. She began offering retreats for inner healing but, admittedly, was not fully prepared to assists those who attended. During her initial retreats, Flora was not equipped in prayer and lacked knowledge about the slow, complex process of full healing. The total person must be ministered to in order for holistic healing to occur.

Wounded people, superficially cured, are not healthy individuals. They have a 'band-aid' on their wounds. Their draining wounds are covered with a dressing; these individuals are like time bombs ready to explode. They need someone anointed by God and trained in pastoral care, a Christian counselor, or a trained lay person who is equipped and anointed, to help them through the healing process. Healing by divine intervention can happen suddenly or miraculously; other times the individuals may need a coach or mentor to assist them in receiving their deliverance. After being released from traumatic relationships, environmental pain and sufferings, the bleeding and draining wounds must dry up. It is very important to have a mentor, pastor, or Christian counselor who will help with the recovery, renewal, and restoration stages.

A young woman was brought to my office because she was contemplating suicide. Her friend brought her to me so that I could pray for her. Sad and despondent, this troubled woman raised the question, "What do I have to live for?" Her friend's response: "You have your family to live for!" The mind is the battleground for spiritual warfare. The woman had been rehearsing over and over in her mind that she had nothing to live for, but she was not bold enough to commit the act of ending her life. She no longer felt as if she was loved or needed by her family; and so the adversary did not pass up this opportunity to bombard her with reasons for not living any longer. She had a needy daughter along with grandchildren, who were dependent on her to help support them. Escapism through suicide is not an option for a Christian; for after death there is judgment.

After praying with her to pull down the walls of defense that had been erected, the young woman fell under the power of God and lay in the Lord's presence for about fifteen minutes before getting up from the floor. I then led her in the prayer of repentance. She asked God to forgive her for meditating upon the thoughts of suicide, for she knew suicide was against the Word of God. Along with receiving God's forgiveness, she rededicated her heart unto the Lord, confessing that her heart had been divided, that she had not had a personal relationship with God. She confessed that feelings of isolation, rejection, and being trapped by circumstances had brought on the suicidal thoughts.

Therefore, I took authority over the thoughts she had been thinking and stressed the importance of having daily fellowship with the Lord through meditating on His Word; through prayer; through praise and worship. She was encouraged to position herself around others who could continue to assist her through to full recovery; to this she agreed. She visited our church on that following Sunday to worship. She entered in smiling while walking down the aisle with her grandchild in tow, as if she was an over-comer! We have not seen her again but we do know that she is still alive—thanks be to God Almighty!

Allow me to expound on her situation: Engaging her in further conversation, I discovered that, as a child, she had been fondled by various males multiple times. She had held onto the hurt, shame, guilt, and anger for over thirty years—not revealing her pain to any other person. She was made to feel ashamed and guilty. Isolation set in because she had been violated, and there was no individual in whom she felt she could confide. Holding on to unforgiveness caused her to become very bitter toward her perpetrators. For her to receive healing, I explained that it was necessary that she allow what she had suppressed for so long to surface in order to forgive each of her violators. She declared that it was not possible for her to forgive them; and to this I assured her that it would take the Lord Jesus to help (and He would)! With His help—along with counseling—she could do it. We then prayed again and asked the Lord to help her to forgive all her abusers.

The process of inner healing, which is the healing of the soul, had just begun. She wept and continued to open up and talk about issues that she had never revealed to others. It is a process for some . . . and in her case years of abuse and suffering from mental breakdowns and demonic attacks would necessitate a certain recovery process. She previously had been under the care of a psychiatrist who treated her medically; but remember, medication is a superficial 'band-aid' for deep wounds that need spiritual healing.

When there are deep wounds, counseling is needed by a pastor, a Christian counselor, or another who is gifted and trained to help the wounded receive their deliverance and healing. When a pastor, spiritual leader, or Christian counselor discerns there is an internal problem, it should be dealt with before it escalates. It is important to have someone empowered or gifted in that area to see the individual through the various stages of healing. Those who are gifted with the prophetic mantle have divine ability to discern certain past issues in a person's life. Speaking it out prophetically may begin the process of deliverance—they realize it is no longer hidden. Some folk get delivered at that moment when they are exhorted to let it go . . . some fall under the power of God and get up a new person! We have seen it happen in our ministry numerous times. The Holy Spirit does a cleansing for those who yield when prayed for; and this happens because they are lying in the presence and under the power of God. Under the shadow of the Almighty is the place to be for miraculous recovery.

In *Release,* the following three major stages of healing have been identified by Flora Slosson Wuellner: spiritual recovery, restoration and renewal. Wuellner experienced major surgery, and the stages of healing were revealed to her during this time. She goes on to explain: "This process of full healing from the experience became for me a fascinating metaphor for the healings on all the levels of body, emotions, and spirit. The first phase, recovery, was the closing of the surgical wound; first in the deep organs and muscles of the body, then the surface layers. In about six weeks, I was pronounced medically recovered, wound closed, no infection, pain gone, and mobility returned."

Wuellner continues, "But this was just the first stage... to my surprise. Now the restoration began. To be restored means to be returned to our former self and to the normal healthy condition that we experienced before the medical problem and the surgical intervention. Medically, I was recovered, but I still needed a lot of rest because of fatigue, toning up the muscles again with gentle exercise; flushing out the toxic residue of drugs and medication."

Wuellner realized "emotional restoration was needed also. I needed time to assimilate, to integrate the experience, to recover my inner balance. I needed time to think over the memories of the experience—the strange things, the funny things, the mystery of it all. Some memories I could share with others; some would move quietly into my private heart."

Lastly, Wuellner explains the renewal stage: "Renewal means to be made fresh. It means a new beginning rather than just returning to the same old ways. As body and spirit recovered and were restored, I began to see more fully the significance of the recent weeks for my whole life. Fresh energy welled up in me. I was learning new ways to live in and with my body, new ways to share what I learned through my ministry." This may be useful in assisting someone without any medical knowledge to understand the process of healing.

I worked in surgery for a brief time during my nursing career and I can recall watching the surgeon open up an area on the body with scalpels, while holding the tissue back with clamps. The blood was suctioned out of the cavity and also large sterile cloth sponges were used to wipe away blood that kept seeping into the wound, because the surgeon had to be able to clearly see what he was attempting to remove. After removing the tumor, organ—or whatever the case may be—it was time to close the wound. The healing process can begin if and when all of the foreign tissue or diseased organ has been removed. Also, healing begins if bacteria have not been introduced into the wound. If these variables do not intervene, the wound will heal from the inside out. When the surgeon realizes there is a problem that has intercepted the healing process, it becomes necessary to get to the root of the problem so as to eradicate it for complete healing to occur.

For inner healing to occur in the soul of the individual it is necessary to go deep into the past to search out things that have been suppressed (pressed down by force). Each emotional wound has to be treated until healing is manifested. People have different ways of dealing with inner pain and suffering; sometimes denial is revealed. Denial is a powerful defense mechanism to avoid painful experiences. You will know when you are delivered because you will be able discuss to it freely, or forgive and release those responsible for wounding you.

There are various numbers who have sustained emotional, mental, and spiritual injuries—individuals who have been injured in feelings and sensibilities. Their injury may have happened through some form of abuse be it sexual, emotional, or physical. The individual is left to deal with issues that will eventually become problematic. Truly, people are bleeding on the inside with only a 'band-aid' as a dressing. The 'band-aid' they use to cover up the hurt may be in their use of street drugs or prescription medication. They may engage in alcoholic or eating binges, or overindulge in certain activities to help them forget the past; however, the issue needs to be dealt with so that the one in bondage can be set free.

There needs to be an anointed mentor to cut into the deepest infected area to clean out the wound for total healing. Jesus came to heal the broken hearted and He is still operating in healing today, using men and women mightily. "*How God anointed Jesus of Nazareth with the Holy Ghost and with power, who went about doing good, and healing all that were oppressed of the devil; for God was with* Him" (Acts 10:38).

Pastors, spiritual leaders, and Christian counselors are called to heal the brokenhearted. Sometimes it is the weight of sin, such as unforgiveness, that weighs a person down and they cannot get what they need through secular counseling. As spiritual leaders or counselors, we assess and evaluate for the strongholds that are oppressing them, so that a successful strategy can be utilized to assist with their deliverance. There is always a probability that deliverance from demonic strongholds may be necessary.

The walking wounded ask, "Who can I trust to tell what I am really going through? When I discover someone to assist me, can I trust them to not reveal my story to someone else? Will they take advantage of me? I know confession is a risk that must be taken in order to receive my inner healing, but can I trust you?" Pray and ask the Holy Spirit for guidance. God has prepared someone to assist you through your healing process. It is time for the captive to be set free. People have a tendency to live their lives in hypocrisy; they smile on the outside, but the inside is usually broken and hurting. The 'band-aid' must come off in order to deal with the deep issues of the past and present. Make a decision to be healed from the inside to the outside—no more superficial, shallow, or surface healing of deeply buried wounds!

What significance is there in forgiving another? For one thing it allows you to be forgiven by the Lord Jesus; for as we forgive others, we are forgiven. Jesus taught His disciples about the benefit of forgiving others:

> *And whenever you stand praying, if you have anything against anyone, forgive him and let it drop (leave it, let it go), in order that your Father who is in heaven may also forgive you your (own) failings and shortcomings and let them drop. But if you do not forgive, neither will your Father in heaven forgive your failings and shortcomings* (Mark 11:25, 26 AMP).

I believe that forgiveness is one key to receiving inner healing. In our ministry we have prayed for people and the power of God was manifested so, that they fell under the power of the Holy Spirit. When they got up their entire countenance was changed because of the anointing. God had delivered them and made them whole.

I address now this issue of offense: Some people become offended and later emotionally wounded as a result of holding onto a grudge. The verb *offend* means to commit a sin or crime, to hurt the feelings of another or to create resentment and anger toward someone; to annoy, affront or bother. I pray this will help pastors, spiritual leaders, and others who are confronted often with this issue.

There are some individuals who easily become offended, that is, angry, insulted or provoked; they will usually run rather than try to bring about some resolution to the problem.

A brother offended is harder to be won over than a strong city, and [their] contentions separate them like the bars of a castle (Proverbs 18:19 AMP).

An offended person will strike back by sowing seeds of discord, to bring relief to their perceived hurt, before he or she leaves a church, ministry or a place of employment. Their aim is to strike back and hurt the way they believed someone has hurt them; and the more they dwell on the insult the larger it becomes. Usually old wounds that have been superficially healed will feed on the offense and start draining again. Emotional issues such as unforgiveness, resentment, bitterness, and hatred will surface and cause internal and communal hemorrhaging; it then is important to allow the purging or hemorrhaging to be free to flow from deep wounds. Be an excellent listener—serious issues are flowing out of their inner person.

You are there to listen and intervene through the power of the Holy Spirit. You are purposed to assist them in getting their deliverance from demonic invasion, spiritual brokenness, emotional wounds, and from soul ties. Lay hands on, rebuke and bind any demonic strongholds; cast them out to dry places; pray the prayer of faith over them, then loose the anointing of the Holy Spirit to penetrate and saturate them. As stated previously, individuals sometimes fall under the power of God and while lying in His presence are totally transformed. Others may need a series of counseling sessions. Most importantly, you allow the Word of God to transform your life.

How can one be delivered or receive deep spiritual transformation or inner healing from these issues? As previously stated, transformation and healing begin by confessing there is a problem and by allowing guilt and shame of past experiences to surface so they can be dealt with. Each issue is confronted in order for the individual involved to become free. John the Baptist proclaimed that it is important to "repent" or "think differently; that is, change your mind, regretting your sins and changing your conduct" (Matthew 3:2). This is the first step to receiving Jesus as Savior and Lord.

Many times, individuals who have issues with boldly addressing or discussing a situation that has arisen will run and create communal problems; they run to and fro, becoming spiritual vagabonds. A vagabond is one who moves from one place to another, a shiftless irresponsible person. These individuals always feel they are the ones that are right, that others are wrong or have mistreated them; therefore, they cause havoc, ruin, and destruction because they have not been delivered from the perceived offense. They come in with a 'band-aid' over their hurts, just like a small child does when he or she is wounded. A crying child can be soothed with that 'band-aid' but, in some instances, an internally-wounded individual only feels better when he or she wounds someone else.

Do you remember injuring yourself as a small child and once a 'band-aid' was applied to the injury, you suddenly forgot the pain? You ceased crying and once again proceeded to engage in play activities. With spiritually and emotionally-wounded people who allow hurt, anger, offense, or injury to seep into their inner self, wounds created become so deeply buried that it takes a miracle from God to deliver and make them whole again. Those wounded may need guidance in seeing their need for a loving, caring person who will assist them through their deliverance process. I do mean assist; for the wounded individual has to desire that a transformation takes place in their lives!

As a pastor, I have witnessed an offended person shift from place to place, never growing enough roots anywhere to accomplish anything. Some uproot themselves during times of trials; they do not understand that God allows adversity in all of our lives to build character in us for His kingdom's sake. Their place of pain would be their place of gain if they endured the trial or temptation . . . God is trying to bring stability to their lives.

At various times, I have seen some individuals angrily leave a church or ministry and then enter another place looking for acceptance. What caused their departure could well have been an opportunity for them to be used by God, by humbly and optimistically confronting the offender to bring about a resolution to the offense. Yet there was no vision past the inner pain and suffering they felt. Often, individuals in conflict are blinded to the fact that God does allow trials to perfect some things that concern us. Anger may not have been shown at the other ministry initially; but remember that before leaving the other church, they created havoc or ruin because they had not been delivered—neither had they since exiting the last ministry. The person left wounded but healed superficially.

In other words their wounds were camouflaged; they were able to hide or cover up their wounds with false humility, laughter, attire, and even possibly over friendliness—therefore superficially healed. Discord may have been sown previously . . . leaders may have been more than likely discredited . . . and others may have been partakers of this person's sins. Wounded people will eventually wound other people because of their pain and hurt.

Now this new ministry is just what they have been looking for to prove their competence and value; especially if it is a newly planted church or one they perceive will need and use their talents, gifts, and calling. They do not realize that whatever the offense was that caused their departure from that earlier fellowship will eventually happen again. Satan stirs discord among brothers and sisters; sometimes the old nature in a person will surface time and time again. And God also tests His sons and daughters! Such individuals are blind to their own character flaws; they are not healed from past hurts, and they have applied 'band-aids' over their wounds.

The 'band-aid' may represent agreement, acceptance or consolation. Many times, the desire not to offend will cause a person to agree with someone who has come to them for help. Pastors and leaders have a tendency to compromise, instead of speaking the truth in love. A ministry may, initially, allow a wounded person to work in the church because there is a need; but this creates a temporary 'band-aid' there is still the root problem that needs to be addressed, as it relates to internal issues. Eventually a wounded person is given some responsibility, without proper training, because they have manipulated their way in . . . and as a leader you have become emotionally involved, without discussing the real issue. A small church is often so elated to welcome new members that its pastor may overlook things initially discerned; this discernment could be a warning to avoid later problems.

Consider the following example: A young woman joined our church in the 90's who was not faithful, but caused havoc, because she felt her gifts were not being recognized and utilized. She had just come in from a lifestyle of night clubbing and riotous living and, being a babe in Christ, knew nothing about how to live as a Christian. I believe she left the church and returned more than once . . . but she did not have a teachable spirit.

In 2008, she returned to inform me that she had been called into the ministry and was anointed. She said, "The anointing that is on my life causes a lot of spiritual leaders to be jealous of me. I am not accepted by pastors because they are intimidated when I am around." I observed her and realized that she was not humble and had not been taught how to conduct herself as a minister under spiritual leadership. She boasted about herself and exhibited a "taking over" spirit. She called herself a prophetess but there was no prophetic order about her; and, again, she did not have a teachable spirit. She left our church when I and another elder confronted her in love concerning her behavior—defined by boasting, aggressiveness, domination, and taking quick offence. She denied it all and proceeded to declare that everywhere she goes, the pastors are jealous of her anointing.

I had an inward witness that this young lady was not going to be receptive to work under leadership. We tried to discuss how we could help her and her response was to become emotional: She cried, spewed accusations, and became so defensive that we were unable to assist her. She repeatedly discredited leadership in the various churches she had been affiliated with and refused to listen as we tried to discuss the issues we observed during the short time she was with us. Had she been willing to sit and listen, it could have possibly worked out for her; however, she left our church and later had problems at other churches.

In the spring of 2010, I saw her at a shopping mall and she then informed me that a pastor had ordained her and that she was preaching. Prayerfully, she has received her deliverance and inner healing that was so much needed. She was wounded from what she perceives as rejection; therefore, she will eventually wound others because she has not dealt with past hurts, even from childhood.

This is an example of an emotionally wounded person who needs inner healing before trying to lead others. It reminds me of a surgical wound I had to evaluate in 2009: I knew from the moment it was assessed that there were going to be problems. The wound was draining, swollen, warm and slightly redden, with a non-healing look about it that indicated it was more than likely infected. I made the initial visit to admit the patient into our healthcare services, but someone else was responsible for her daily wound care.

I discovered that upon my return to her home, approximately two weeks later, her wound had to be reopened by the surgeon because of infection from the initial surgery. The abdominal wound that was reopened was larger than my fist. Bacteria had entered the wound from either an internal or external source. The 'band-aid' was the stay sutures that had initially been put in place to secure the incision while the infection was seething deep within the wound. Regardless of bandages, whenever there is an infection, it will find a way to drain.

God made the body complete with intricate physiological details to alert one of impending issues. A healthy wound will not be discolored, nor grow hot with fever; it will not drain yellow or green drainage, nor have a foul smell. It is the same way with a healthy person: She or he will not spew out venom or poison; entertain malicious gossip; curse or slander, nor discredit; hold unforgiveness or bitterness; compete with or be jealous of, nor be happy about the misfortunes of another.

Just as the surgeon must immediately correct an infected surgical wound, so should the emotionally wounded be delivered and healed before taking a leadership position in a church or a managerial position for a company. It is wise to find out why a person is no longer volunteering or employed by a ministry or business. Ask questions about their former church or other place of employment; inquire into their relationship with their former boss or church leader. If they left offended, they will eventually speak something to discredit their former leader. Do not be quick to fill positions without finding out the character of the person who is to fill the office.

Wounded people wound other people—sometimes to the point of being hopeless. As pastors we are responsible to be overseers of God's church. We are called to be good stewards of His estate and to not allow people, harboring different spirits, to manipulate their way in to speak over and touch His sheep. What God entrusts to His pastors is not to be taken lightly! Apostle Peter admonishes spiritual leaders and I agree with the Word of God:

> *The elders which are among you I exhort, who am also an elder, and a witness of the sufferings of Christ, and also a partaker of the glory that shall be revealed. Feed the flock of God which is among you, taking the oversight thereof, not by constraint, but willingly, not for filthy lucre, but of a ready mind; neither as being lords over God's heritage, but being examples to the flock* (1 Peter 5:1-3).

There are different ways that a person can sustain inner wounds; some are wounded by situations out of their control, while others are wounded by those who deliberately seek to inflict pain, be it emotional, mental or physical damage. A woman unable to bear children may experience certain emotional issues such as, shame, sorrow, anger, and self-condemnation.

A woman I knew from my childhood would dress in clothes worn by pregnant women; for she believed herself to be or pretended to be pregnant. Sometimes the state of a person can become so delusional that they may be diagnosed as psychotic. Mental-emotional depression can be the result of an unfilled expectation. I do not think this certain lady was able to have children. She was barren and was acting out an unfulfilled desire.

When an individual is overcome or consumed by a depressed state, it is not easily overcome by confession. This individual does not believe that God can help them. It may take sessions of counseling, prayer, and deliverance for them to be released from the stronghold of a spirit of heaviness. Some people may have to be medicated for various reasons, which is the reason we have physicians and pharmaceutical products. For whatever situation you are in, there is help available.

In 1st Samuel the story is told of an Israelite named Elkanah who had two wives; one was fruitful in bearing him children and the other unable to bear, for she was barren. Peninnah bore children, but Hannah could not because the Lord had closed her womb. Peninnah would provoke Hannah, to upset and anger her over the fact that the Lord had closed her womb; thus, Hannah sustained repeated insults from her rival. The Book of Samuel does not say Hannah was ashamed or depressed, but her described behaviors, such as, a loss of appetite and crying suggests so. In the Hebrew culture it was disgraceful to be unable to bear children. It was also the custom of the day to have more than one wife. This was not God's perfect will but it did happen and, oftentimes, was the root of unhappiness in the family.

Elkanah, his wives and children would travel annually to Shiloh to worship and sacrifice to the Lord. Elkanah loved Hannah and would therefore give a double portion to her for the sacrifice. In spite of her husband's love, Hannah cried and would not eat during the journey to Shiloh, fretting because of her barrenness. She had to sit in the company of her enemy Peninnah, who could bear children by Hannah's husband, and be taunted.

Elkanah wanted to know why Hannah was sad. He asked her, "Am I not better than ten sons?" I believe that she felt ashamed. This is a coinciding thought posited by Dr. Edward P. Wimberly in his book, *In Moving from Shame to Self-Worth:* "Devastating shame blocks people's ability to discern a caring God. They need to spend time in a mediating relationship with some caring others before they can entertain the notion that God or Jesus could actually care for them." Dr. Wimberly underscores that in a particular case it took two years for shame to be sufficiently neutralized before one counselee could discuss God and Jesus in relationship to herself.

Elkanah expressed his love to Hannah; yet she had to endure Peninnah tearing, harassing, or lacerating her emotions whenever they were together. Peninnah had sons and daughters and Hannah had none. It may not have been the inability to bear children that hurt Hannah the most; possibly it was the continuous insults from Peninnah that repeatedly wounded her emotionally. Remember, Dr. Wimberly points out that "a person with shame believes that they are flawed and unlovable." Even if in caring and loving relationships, such individuals need time to believe that God or someone else can love them.

In some cases pastoral counseling is necessary. When served by a spirit-filled counselor who is anointed to pray, there will be favorable results when that intercessor earnestly seeks the Lord for His desire, and prays accordingly. God can miraculously deliver an individual when they cry out for help, and one blessed with the mantle of deliverance may assist in bringing release to a person who is suffering emotionally. Once again, there are times when it takes another person to assist an individual in understanding how to shift their attention to something that is a positive note in their lives.

Hannah's husband loved her and it did not matter to him that she was barren. Sometimes, it is difficult for people to accept genuine love from another . . . if they hold on to feelings of worthlessness. Even if Hannah never bore children, her husband loved her for who she was. He did not love the second wife as much as he did Hannah; it appears he tolerated her and she was a means for procreation. God created Adam, and later Eve, and gave them instructions for replenishing the earth:

> *And God blessed them, and God said unto them, Be fruitful, and multiply, and replenish the earth, and subdue it; and have dominion over the fish of the sea, and the fowl of the air, and over every living thing that moves upon the earth* (Genesis 1:28).

Hannah received counseling from Eli the priest at the temple in Shiloh. Eli initially thought she was drinking wine because of her outbursts of pain. Inwardly, she was bleeding: sorrow, painful memories, low self-worth, and feelings of failure were the reason for her outbursts. Hannah was the one suffering and to the degree that she needed consolation, her husband could not console her. Elkanah could not identify with the hurts of a woman who could not bear children because he had never been (nor would be) in that role. He fulfilled the role of a parent by creating children with another—Peninnah, who bore him sons and daughters. Although it was the culture of that time, there were unresolved issues among the wives. Even during times of tolerance, there must have been communal "sickness and deep wounds" that needed inner healing.

Elkanah loved Hannah and only tolerated Peninnah for her child-bearing and child-rearing abilities; therefore, jealously was likely one issue that arose. Jealously is a stronghold that is responsible for causing a person to hurt others; it is a spirit that seeks to destroy relationships. It is a spirit that causes one to murder another physically, emotionally, mentally, and spiritually. These are some of the signs and symptoms of a jealous spirit: envy, resentment, an overbearing attitude, rebellion, hatred, bitterness, pride, strife, contention, and sowing discord.

Spiritual counseling and deliverance will more than likely have to occur before an individual can be released from a jealousy stronghold. It is necessary to confess one's faults to another to receive help while in the process of deliverance. The Word of God says, "*Confess your trespasses* (faults) *to one another, and pray for one another, that you may be healed. The effective, fervent prayer of the righteous avails much*" (James 5:16).

Dr. Francis MacNutt makes the following observation in his work, *The Power to Heal:* "The need for inner healing usually comes forth in tears that have often been left uncried for many years. If we minister with that person for a time, the inner healing takes place, usually in an easier way than when the power of the Spirit is not as manifestly present. Occasionally, if evil spirits are present, the power of the Spirit stirs them up; they can't stand that degree of the power of the Spirit, so they surface." Dr. MacNutt continues by stating, "Again, when this happens, we can take the person to a place where we have the privacy to minister and finish the deliverance. In short, anything which is not simple and peaceful is not direct action of the Spirit, but is the reaction of wounded human nature or the forces of evil."

Dr. MacNutt discusses signs and symptoms that alert the one praying for a person who needs inner healing, which appear in the shedding of tears, or some emotional eruption. I agree, for many times while praying for others, I have witnessed them beginning to cry, sometimes silently. At those times, you are able to discern hidden hurt that is unresolved; and when you then minister to their inner pain, it results in their deliverance after a period of time. Again, some may fall under the power of the Spirit and receive their deliverance while lying in the presence of God.

Sometimes, deliverance may take longer if there is a demonic force present and it refuses to release the person. The evil force cannot stand in the presence of the Holy Spirit; it has to go. When we first began ministering deliverance, it took us some time to discern an evil force from a wounded spirit. If you are not seasoned in deliverance, you may think all negative reactions are caused by an evil spirit; however, one's spirit can be wounded from losses, a divorce, sickness, or any assault you cannot obtain victory over.

For instance, in the Book of Ruth, the loss of Naomi's husband and her two sons resulted in her being wounded, and ultimately bitter. Repeated losses, and other surrounding circumstances, can wound your spirit. Naomi lost her family and also her means of financial survival. She was thoroughly depressed when she returned to her homeland; she expressed no joy in life because she had suffered significant losses. One assault after another made it difficult to overcome the repeated insults. This is the reason it is important to be connected to others who can minister to you if tragedy should occur.

In *Counseling Through Your Bible Handbook*, June Hunt explains that "Bitterness is a major cause of depression." She then asks, "Are you repressing anger over the loss of... a loved one, expectations, self-esteem, respect for others, control, health or abilities, possessions, personal goals? If so, read Ephesians 4:31: "*Get rid of all bitterness, rage, and anger, brawling and slander, along with every form of malice*." (p. 125) Hunt goes on to ask specifically: "Are you internalizing stress over . . . work difficulties, financial obligations, relocation, family responsibilities, marital problems, troubled child, workload, alcoholic spouse? If so, read 1 Peter 5:7: *"Cast all your anxiety on Him because He cares for you."* Even our deep disappointments must be resolved or our bitterness will cause trouble. Unresolved anger and bitterness can hurt those who are close to us." (p. 126)

Joan Hunt gives valuable insight on what can defeat depression since bitterness is one of its major causes. She poses a third question and its answer: "What can help defeat depression? Allow the light of God's love to permeate your ditch of darkness and guide you to the road to transformation." Hunt then offers the following steps one should use to C.O.N.Q.U.E.R depression:

C- Confront any loss in your life, allowing yourself to grieve and be healed. "[*There is*] *a time to weep and a time to laugh, a time to mourn and a time to dance"* (Ecclesiastes 3:4).

O- Offer your heart to God for cleansing and confess your sins. *"If we claim to be without sin, we deceive ourselves and the truth is not in us. If we confess our sins, He is faithful and just and will forgive us our sins and purify us from all unrighteousness*" (I John 1:8, 9).

N- Nurture thoughts that focus on God's great love for you. "*I have loved you with an everlasting love; I have drawn you with loving kindness"* (Jeremiah 31:3).

Q- Quit negative thinking and negative self-talk. "*Whatever is true, whatever is noble, whatever is right, whatever is pure, whatever is lovely, whatever is admirable—if anything is excellent or praiseworthy—think about these things*" (Philippians 4:8).

U- Understand God's eternal purpose for allowing personal loss and heartache. *"We know that all things work for the good of those who love Him, who have been called according to his purpose"* (Romans 8:28).

E- Exchange your hurt and anger for thanksgiving, and give thanks even when you don't feel thankful. "*Give thanks in all circumstances; for this is God's will for you in Christ Jesus"*(*1Thessalonians* 5:18).

R- Remember that God is sovereign over your life, and He promises hope for your future. "*For you have been my hope, O Sovereign Lord, my confidence since my youth"*

(Psalm 71:5). (All Scriptures quoted by June Hunt are taken from the NIV Bible.)

The Book of Job is about a man who had everything and lost all he had, except a wife who spoke derogatorily against God. Job's wife challenged God. "*Are you still holding on to your integrity? Curse God and die!*" Job replied, "*You are talking like a foolish woman. Shall we accept good from God, and not trouble?*" *In all this, Job did not sin in what he said*" (Job 2:9, 10 NIV). Job suffered the devastating loss of his children, live-stock, servants, and health; and he made some mistakes in words and attitude while he endured the suffering. In all his suffering Job humbled himself, repented to God, and prayed for his friends because of their presumptuous words; their accusations indicated that Job had sinned, that God was punishing him. Job passed the test of the accuser Satan, because he did not turn against God. After Job had prayed for his friends, the Lord allowed him to become more prosperous than before; God gave him twice as much as he had before the temporary losses in Job 42:10.

Here is one person's poignant statement about her deliverance and healing from inner suffering in MacNutt's *The Power to Heal*: "And now to feel so light and free; freer than the birds singing with crazy versatility, just outside my window. More joyful than the song they were singing, happy to be alive, so happy, no longer having to pretend . . . just free to be me, free to move around, and most of all free to love everyone, especially those I live with. What an exhilarating experience of being once more with Jesus."

This is one way you will know that you are delivered: There will be a freedom that has not been experienced before, or for a long time. There is an undeniable release of weights and pressures when deliverance occurs. You will see things from a different perspective; there will not be a fear of being overcome again by previous experiences. Things that you wanted to do but were fearful to venture out on will arise again, and you will go forth with purpose guiding you. You will declare that this is not your season to fail. Inner healing many times may also result in a person receiving their physical healing. Those made free by Christ Jesus are free indeed.

Emotional eating causes physical illness because it is usually careless, spur of the moment, unprepared diets—loaded with sugar, starch, chocolate, caffeine, grease and sodium. Consuming large quantities to feel better emotionally can lead to hypertension, diabetes, high cholesterol, obesity, heart failure, strokes, and other medical problems. I emotionally consumed food for years and I was also an emotional shopper; it made me feel better to be able to ease my hurt or rejection with food or shopping.

All my life I have eaten what I desired, until I began to have problems with my blood pressure. As a nurse, I knew better but still did not practice discipline. As children, we were reared to eat what we wanted and homemade dessert was available daily; a cake baked in our home would only last one evening. There were few restrictions on our eating. I believe this to be our grandmother's compensation for other things we lacked as children. We did not have the amenities enjoyed by some with whom we were associated because our dad did not provide for us. As a child I was overweight, and I have struggled with my weight all my life. I realize now that eating when I was not hungry was satisfying another need, now a persistent issue for years.

The observed elevation in my blood pressure has prompted me to eat more wisely, by using less sodium, reducing the fat and cholesterol in my diet, and enjoying more vegetables and fresh fruit. I use the *Ms. Dash* product and check all ingredients for their sodium content. Additionally, I have joined the YMCA to be a part of a regular exercise program. Anxiety can be channeled into something constructive, such as praying, praising and worshiping God; meditating on God's Word; helping someone else who is less fortunate, or volunteering in a community organization. We are not to worry or be anxious about anything: "*Do not fret or have any anxiety about anything, but in every circumstance and in everything, by prayer and petition* (definite requests), *with thanksgiving, continue to make your wants known to God*" (Philippians 4:6 AMP).

PRAYER FOR DELIVERANCE AND HEALING

Father, in the name of Jesus, I come to you in need of deliverance from sin, self, and Satan. I ask You to forgive me for my involvement in any sins I have committed. Forgive me, save me, and accept me as your son or daughter. I believe that Jesus died for my sins, that is, He took on all of my sins on the cross. I accept what He has done for me while on the cross. I know that I do not have to be sin or guilt ridden anymore; Jesus has declared me not guilty. All I have to do is believe in my heart and confess with my mouth that Jesus is the Son of God, and that God has raised Him from the dead, through the power of the Holy Spirit.

> *That if you confess with your mouth the Lord Jesus, and believe in your heart that God has raised Him from the dead; you shall be saved. For with the heart one believes unto righteousness, and with the mouth confession is made unto salvation* (Romans 10:9, 10 NIV).

I believe and confess the Lord Jesus as Savior and Lord of my life. I renounce every generational curse that has come upon my life for four generations. Name them:

_________________________. _________________________.
_________________________.
_________________________. _________________________.
_________________________.

I repent; that is, I ask the Lord to forgive me for not calling on the name of Jesus to save me. I call on your name now Jesus and ask that You come into my heart to save me. You said in your Word, Lord, "*. . . Everyone who calls on the name of the Lord will be saved* (Romans 10:13 NIV).. Jesus has given the church authority, that is, keys to use in His behalf to render the devil and his demons powerless:

> *I will give you the keys of the kingdom of heaven; and whatever you bind* (declare to be improper and unlawful) *on earth must be what is already bound in heaven; and whatever you loose* (declare lawful) *on earth must be what is already loosed in heave*n (Matthew 16:19 AMP).

For example, I bind the spirit of fear, in the name of Jesus, and send it to the dry places. I declare it is powerless and ineffective against me. I loose power, love, and a sound mind, in Jesus' name.

Lord, with Your help I forgive each person who has hurt me (name them one by one if possible), and release them. I make a commitment to read the Word of God; to meditate upon it; to pray it, and live it daily. I declare and decree that generational curses that have been in my family will not come on me or my seed. Your Word, Lord, will be a lamp unto my feet and a light unto my path, in the name of Jesus. I praise the Lord for my liberty!

A generational curse may be, for example, a perverse spirit that engages in all forms of sexual immorality. It could be a spirit of lying, or a familiar spirit that engages in witchcraft, voodoo, magic, curses, fortune telling, palm reading or hypnotism. Some other generational curses may be poverty, or certain ailments under the spirit of infirmity, such as: heart disease, high blood pressure, and asthma. It is important to know too that if you want deliverance, you need to see yourself delivered . . . repent . . . renounce the curse you are under through generational ties, and confess the Word of God.

You may need a coach or mentor to assist you with your deliverance; if so, expect to be set free. Study and confess the Word of God daily for your healing, i.e. "*I have already been healed by His stripes . . . .*" (cf. 1 Peter 2:24; Isaiah 53:5). Confess the Word of God: "*Greater is He in me than He that is in the world*" (1 John 4:4). Be assured of God's truth: "*Now this is the confidence that we have in Him, that if we ask anything according to His will, He hears us. And if we know that He hears us, whatever we ask, we know that we have the petitions that we have asked of Him*" (1 John 5:14, 15 NKJV).

Wounded people must be healed from the inside to fully recover. It may take sessions of counseling and prayer to be set free, but do not give up. There are those who are committed to assisting others in receiving their deliverance and healing. God desires for you to be free; therefore, He has the right coach or mentor for you. When you are wounded, do not cover up the wounds; confront individuals in love, tell them how you feel. Let them know you were hurt when certain things were spoken to you. Forgive those you believed have hurt you. Continue to work on it if you are struggling with forgiving someone. I have struggled at times in my life with forgiveness. Even today, if I come under heated fire by someone's tongue, I find myself saying, "I will be better, not bitter." Yes, I have to work on it; it does not just happen.

You might be surprised to find out some people do not realize they have offended others in the past. An offended one may carry a grudge for years; sometimes the person offended is in bondage but the other is free. You may ask, "How can this be?" The person(s) did not realize they had offended you by something they said or did. While they have moved on with their life, you remain resentful and bitter. Unforgiveness dries up the bone marrow, making them brittle, and is thought to be partly responsible for arthritis. So deal with it!—the price is not worth it. Get on your knees—cry out to God to help you forgive and release the individual(s)! God is a very present help in your time of need . . . and He is merciful, even when we do not deserve it. Do not allow old wounds to be covered with a 'band-aid'; allow instead the penetrating power of God's Word and worship to infiltrate and eradicate old memories, thoughts, feelings, and wounds of past experiences.

You must understand how significant and powerful the Word of God is; consider the Amplified Version of Hebrews 4:12:

> *For the Word that God speaks is alive and full of power [making it active, operative, energizing, and effective]; it is sharper than any two-edged sword, penetrating to the dividing line of the breath of life (soul) and[the immortal] spirit, and of joints and marrow [of the deepest parts of our nature],*

exposing and sifting and analyzing and judging the very thoughts and purposes of the heart.

David cried out to the Lord in his distress and God heard him. Psalm 86 is a prayer of David; read and meditate on verses 1-6, again from the Amplified Bible:

Incline your ear, O Lord, and answer me, for I am poor and distressed, needy and desiring. Preserve my life, for I am godly and dedicated; O my God, save Your servant, for I trust in You [leaning and believing on You, committing all and confidently looking to You, without fear or doubt]. Be merciful and gracious to me, O Lord, for to You do I cry all the day. Make me, Your servant, to rejoice, O Lord, for to You do I lift myself up. For You, O Lord, are good, and ready to forgive [our trespasses, sending them away, letting them go completely and forever]; and You are abundant in mercy and loving- kindness to all those who call upon You. Give ear, O Lord, to my prayer; and listen to the cry of my supplications.

David was so confident that God heard him and would answer him accordingly, that he states in verse 7, "*In the day of trouble I will call on You, for you will answer me.*"

God has given us powerful weapons to help us overcome obstacles or cumbersome circumstances, such as His Word, prayer, praise, worship, the name of Jesus, the blood of Jesus, and empowerment by the Holy Spirit. We also have the full armor of God that we must apply daily according to Ephesians 6:11-18. Everything that pertains to life and godliness has been given unto us, sons and daughters of God. It is through our relationship with the Lord Jesus that we inherit such benefits, and through our continual fellowship, communion, and intimacy with the Holy Spirit He reveals more to us, which is a mystery to those who do not confess Jesus as Lord and Savior.

6

WOUNDED WOMEN WOUND OTHER WOMEN

Is there no balm in Gilead? Is there no physician there? Why then is not the health of the daughter of my people restored? [Because Zion {the church}, no longer enjoyed the presence of the Great Physician!] (Jeremiah 8:22 AMP, emphasis added).

Wounded women who wound other women have issues worth addressing, though very painful and at times quite perplexing. Various sources account for this turbulence, ranging from emotional, mental, sexual and physical abuse to disappointments, rejection and perceived failures. Additionally, there is that constant need to accomplish something and be affirmed by others. It also stems from not receiving the love, support, respect, and affection that is needed to be whole.

During my twenty three years in ministry, I have come in contact with wounded women who have not been healed from previous issues of insecurity, shame, rejection, pain, fear, and low self-esteem. These women have a tendency to wound other women. As we study the Scriptures, we discover this to be true from the beginning of recorded time throughout history; there are many relevant examples in the Hebrew Bible.

Women have been subjected to scores of negative conditions from infancy to the stage of adulthood, thus the question: *Is there no healing for God's daughters?* I submit to you that there is indeed healing and restoration for God's daughters. It comes through discerning how to get in the presence of a loving God to find the comfort, love, peace, and acceptance available to us. Through the leading and guiding of the Holy Spirit, who tugs at our heart, we find out that there is a place God has reserved for us that no one else can fill. God does use others to assist us in our time of need, and it is important to know that you are not alone in your sufferings. Once we discover how God longs for us to be made whole, it is then up to us—each individual—to seek Him and to accept the help that is available.

The time to seek the Lord is during your wilderness experience of despair, loneliness, hopelessness and shame. He is your confidant, that is, your close, trusted friend, who will never leave nor forsake you. You may be in a similar place as I was at one time when seeking the Lord was the furthest thing from my mind. I had a mind of my own—thought I could handle whatever came my way, but I was wrong! I tried to hide my failures but this did not work; my issues almost overwhelmed me because pride would not let me seek help, nor call on the Lord. This was also a time when I was void of good, positive, godly role models in my life to help me find my way back to God.

Korah shows us an experienced longing for God in the midst of one's many distresses:

> *As a deer thirsts for streams of water, so I thirst for you, God. I thirst for the living God. Where can I go to meet with him? Day and night, my tears have been my food. People are always saying, 'Where is your God?' When I remember these things, I speak with a broken heart. I used to walk with the crowd and lead them to God's Temple with songs of praise. Why am I so sad? Why am I so upset? I should put my hope in God and keep praising Him, my Savior and my God* (Psalms 42:1-5 NCV).

According to the Hebrew Bible, Korah was an Israelite and a director of music in the temple of the Lord. Offered here is a poignant description of his experience of being cut off from the community of worship . . . feeling distant from God's presence . . . longing for intimacy with the Creator. For the believer who lived during Old Testament times, there was only one place where the true worship of the Lord was possible—the temple in Jerusalem; the Jerusalem Temple was the God-ordained place of worship:

> *Yet I have chosen Jerusalem, that my name may be there, and I have chosen David to be over my people Israel. For now I have chosen and sanctified this house, that my name may be there forever, and my eyes and my heart will be there perpetually* (2 Chronicles 6:6; 7:16 NKJV).

Our heart is the God-ordained place of worship for believers today; this is what we give to God; and this is our meeting place with Him. Proverbs tells us that sickness can be overcome but there is no medicine for a broken spirit: "*A healthy spirit conquers adversity, but what can you do when the spirit is crushed?*" (Proverbs 18:14Msg). It is important to have a personal relationship with Christ in order to overcome adversities; our fellowship with Him is like medicine to fix our problem. "*A merry heart makes a cheerful countenance, but by sorrow of the heart the spirit is broken. A merry heart does good like medicine, but a broken spirit dries the bones*" (Proverbs 15:13; 17:22 NKJV).

Assisting us with our deliverance will be wise men and women who have been prepared by God. We must recognize that not all pastors, all counselors, and all mentors are equipped to help bring deliverance, healing, and restoration to those who need inner healing; some have been equipped as [spiritual] counselors. There is someone God has divinely appointed to assist you in your time of need.

It will take seasoned, mature, skillful, wise, truthful and loving women who have been chosen by God to help heal the broken hearts of some women. A high incidence of incest has occurred and still occurs in families. So many women have been abused by their fathers, brothers, uncles, cousins, as well as pastors and other men whom they trusted; therefore, it may be important for these women to be counseled by another woman because of that very abuse—especially in sexual abuse cases. It is difficult for some women to develop a loving, trusting relationship with men, since the person who was to have provided protection for them is the very one who abused them.

I believe that with a God-appointed and anointed counselor most women will learn to trust again, to develop long lasting relationships. It will take help from women who have been truly empowered by God, who are not afraid to counsel, confront in love, lay hands on, deliver, heal and restore. Most women can empathize with another woman because many have been through the same or similar trials in life. Some would have lost their mind had it not been for the grace of God. We praise the Lord for allowing us to go through and come out with a story to help someone else. Women who are overcomers-it is time for you to be transparent; others need to hear your story! This world is in such turmoil, chaos and confusion is all around your story may just save the life of a adolescent or another woman. We do not always know what God has purposed for us to do until we do it. Each one of us have been allowed to come to this earth with God having a purpose in mind for our lives. Seek Him, you may not yet know your value, but you are valuable.

Women with deep wounds need to know there is hope in the midst of their perceived hopelessness. Take the mask off; someone needs a genuine, sincere, spirit filled, anointed woman of God who is not afraid to disclose her state . . . before her deliverance, to free another sister. Most of us have not been saved all of our lives. God is taking the foolish things to confound the wise: men and women with ridiculously foul, past life-styles are now leading mega ministries. If the grace of God was powerful enough to change them, it can for sure change you. All you have to do is want to change and accept the way that God wants to do it. Reframe from trying to do things the way it is seen through your natural eyes, allow the grace of God to expand your horizon. We need to take God out of our finite box. He is an infinite spiritual being, with no limits and no boundaries, no shackles and no chains. Allow Him to enlarge your territory or your unlimited boundaries. We know that weeping may endure for a season, but after that season is over joy comes to make up for all the pain, shame, losses, and failures.

Unless you are a woman, you cannot fully understand or put yourself in a woman's place to experience similar hurt, pain, shame, rejection, and loss. These experiences are different for a woman because she *is* a woman. You may understand from your mother, sister, wife, daughter, or friend's testimony, but never from the actual experience. As women we have tasted and seen that the Lord is good, and nobody but God could have delivered us from some of the mess we were in.

At the same time, women probably understand more about rejection than anyone.

As previously stated, some females are rejected from their mother's wound, during their growing years, and even in adulthood [simply] because of their gender. What is rejection? *Rejection* is declining or refusing to accept or consider someone. The one being rejected is renounced, denied, discarded, or thrown out—looked down on by others with a condescending attitude (ref. Webster's Dictionary and Thesaurus,].

Some people have grown up in a home where they were devalued or treated differently than the others living in that same home. Maybe you were labeled with a name, such as, "dumb,' "silly," "crazy," "stupid" or "imbecile." These may have been labels your family, teachers, so called friends, and others used to get your attention. These are negative words and they may have made you feel like your life had no value. Even though others may have tried to discredit you, God had nothing to do with it. *"For the Lord will not cast off His people, nor will He forsake His inheritance*" (Psalm 94:14). "*God will not forget His people any more than He will forget Himself*" "*If we endure, we shall reign with Him. If we deny Him, He will also deny us. If we are faithless, He remains faithful; He cannot deny Himself* (2 Timothy 2:12, 13 NKJV).

June Hunt is the founder of "Hope for the Heart," a worldwide biblical counseling ministry serving for more than twenty years. Hunt shares some important concepts about rejection, examining the following: "How does rejection breed rejection? When rejected, a chain reaction can occur that leads to more rejection. Through conscious choices, a cycle becomes a pattern that eventually becomes a way of life. Unless truth is embraced, the cycle broken, and the pattern replaced, rejection will continue to breed rejection."

Hunt goes on to say, "Rejection brings on feelings of worthlessness; feeling worthless brings on self-hate; self-hate incites negative behavior to alleviate the pain, and negative behavior reproduces rejection. When you are rejected, be aware of a tendency to over generalize, assuming that others will reject you. Fearing the worst, you may inadvertently push away your remaining friends to prevent further hurt." People have within themselves the tendency to reject others. Because of our fear of further rejection, a superficial wall is put up as a defense to ward off others who may eventually reject us. In preparing for rejection, a potential recipient may withdraw first to protect from further hurt. Elaborating, Hunt says, "When they respond negatively, you will interpret their reaction as confirmation of your deepest fears. This vicious cycle will lead to a self-fulfilling prophecy and explains the saying, 'Rejection breeds rejection. To stop feeling like a 'reject':

1. Do not assume that one person's opinion reflects everyone's opinion.
2. Do not let one person's negative attitude toward you define you.

3. Realize because Jesus calls you "friend" (see Luke 7:34), you can trust that His love will be with you always.
4. Nurture several friendships, focusing on God's description of how true friends treat one another; a true friend will never reject you. "A true friend loves at all times" (Proverbs 17:17a).

As previously stated, I too felt rejected by my parents—especially by my dad. As a child I did not understand that my mother worked to support us, that being in a home that was safe for us was more important than being in a broken home with a dad who spent his money on riotous living and was abusive to her. My salvation was my paternal grandmother and aunt, who loved and cared for us up until adulthood. My mother and her mother loved us also, but my maternal grandmother had other children she was caring for. Again, my mother was our one source of support; our aunt Norma was also another. With our mother work schedule it was not possible for her to take proper care of us. This was my assumption; until a few years before my grandmother died she said that my dad who was her son did not want us living with our mother. It was probably safer at the time for my mother and for us because he was an abusive alcoholic.

I have come to the conclusion it was God's will for me to be with my maternal grandmother because of the call that was on my life. When I look back over my life I see that it did began during my pre-teen years. I developed a love for God, His people, and in assisting them to advance His Kingdom. I believe it was a divine setup, because my paternal grandmother instilled in us the importance of being holy . . . and even though I rejected some of the things she taught me at a certain phase in my life, those teachings have been so important to my Christian journey.

We spent the summer and the Christmas season with my mother, provided the weather was conducive for traveling. She worked for a family and was away from home often; so our time with her was limited during those seasonal visits. I did not allow this to make me bitter or unapproachable. Our maternal grandmother and aunts assisted with our care when we were not with our mother in Louisville.

There comes a season in your life when you realize that a change is necessary: We have to make a decision to be better and not bitter about life's situations that are out of our control, or even those events that we have some power to change. We have to know that there is help for every issue or situation we encounter; there is a way of escape. I agree with the apostle Paul: "*I have strength for all things in Christ who* empowers me [I am ready for anything and equal to anything through Him who infuses inner strength into me; I am self-sufficient in Christ's sufficiency"] (Philippians 4:13 AMP).

Dr. Virginia Harrison, founder and president of *Kingdom of God Ministries, Incorporated*, holds a doctorate in Christian Education from Faith Christian University and a doctorate in counseling from Florida International Seminary. Her book, "*Let It Go!*" was published in 2010, and I am including a portion of her story with permission from Dr. Harrison. Having met her in 2000, I was familiar with her story, which focused on her separation from her husband and how he persuaded most of the congregation to leave their church, and find a separate place to worship away from Dr. Harrison, taking ninety-eight per cent of the members They were leading the church together at the time, and she was the senior pastor. With the split she was not informed of their new meeting place. Harrison discusses the rejection, hurt, anger, pain, physical suffering, mental anguish and shame she felt over the separation . . . for not only did she lose her spouse, she finally had only one congregant left in her church. She confessed her love for her husband and did not understand how this could have happened.

He later confessed that he could not work with Dr. Harrison after she received her Ph.D., and she admits that she went full speed ahead with the church after graduation, affirming that her husband was right: "I promised God that if He would help me through the dissertation, I would focus on the church, which I did." Though she asked her spouse to return after he left more than once, to try and make the marriage work, but he refused.

From this statement I would surmise that her spouse was possibly jealous of her achievements in completing her doctorates, along with other accomplishments and degrees. They could have worked it out if both were willing to surrender some other things that were important to them. Harrison declared her emotions of anger ranged from mild to extreme: "I experienced mild harm when I didn't cast my cares upon the Lord. The extreme harm came when I allowed the anger to cause bodily harm: a nervous stomach, difficulty in concentrating, trouble sleeping and uncontrollable crying at times; wanting to lash out in anger at anyone who hurt me, and at times wishing those people would die or leave my life completely."

She continues by saying, "I went from notoriety to humiliation in ministry and my personal life; from a very comfortable means of economic resources to very limited resources to possibly returning my car back to the dealership to avoid repossession; from a marriage to no marriage; from activity and action to inactivity; from socializing to solitude and loneliness; . . . most importantly . . . waiting . . . and waiting . . . and more waiting." She said, "I cried, complained and wondered when God would bring me out of the wilderness. The Holy Spirit told me not to complain but to praise God in the midst of my trials. It was difficult, but finally, one day at a time, I experienced praising Jesus above my pain. Even so, I still had challenges leaving my past to move forward with the purpose that I have been placed here on earth."

Dr. Harrison had to let go and allow God to become the focus of her life after the ordeal she suffered; it was not easy and it did not happen overnight. There are some conclusions she had to come to in order to move on with her life, which may also assist you, after some unforeseen challenging circumstances occur in your life.

1. Embrace challenges as opportunities . . . for God's miraculous plan.
2. View failure from a different perspective . . . not all failures mean defeat.
3. Embrace a positive mindset . . . praise God to overcome depression.
4. Be strong during the battle . . . set your affections on things above.
5. Be confident about your gifts and talents.
6. Press forward to accomplish God's plan for your life.
7. Acknowledge your weakness to God (Jehovah El Shaddai).
8. Walking in obedience to God (Jehovah Nissi) brings victory in your life.
9. God (Jehovah Jireh) will protect His children.
10. Maintain a champion mentality . . . a setback is only a setup for a comeback.
11. Stand in faith on the Word of God.
12. Demonstrate resilience in Jesus . . . trials and adversities to build character.

13. Turn your scars into stars . . . when given a lemon turn it into lemonade.
14. Maintain a victor mentality and not a victim mentality.

Jesus suffered while on this earth by the hands of humanity and various systems set up to challenge the plan of God, but He was an overcomer for our victory. He is not foreign to the needs and sufferings of His people.

> *For we do not have a High Priest who is unable to understand and sympathize, and have a shared feeling with our weaknesses, and infirmities, and liability to the assaults of temptation, but One who has been tempted in every respect as we are, yet without sinning* (Hebrews 4:15 AMP).

Jesus understood suffering because He experienced various kinds during His thirty-three years on earth. He also wants you to understand, *"God is our Refuge and Strength [mighty and impenetrable to temptation], a very present and well-proved help in trouble"* (Psalm 46:1 AMP). Even though Jesus suffered and was unjustly treated by others, He refused to walk in unforgiveness.

Jesus warns us to forgive, that we may be forgiven. To do so, the Lord admonishes us, in Mark 11:22, 23, to exercise the God kind of faith, thus being constant and unwavering . . . . If you have this kind of faith, you can speak to situations in your life that may be like a mountain; and when you believe what you say, without doubting, it—whatever it may be—will surely be done. "*For this reason I am telling you, whatever you ask for in prayer, believe* (trust and be confident) *that it is granted to you, and you will get it*" (Mark 11:24 AMP).

> *And whenever you stand praying, if you have anything against anyone, forgive him and let it drop (leave it, let it go), in order that your Father Who is in heaven may also forgive you your [own] failings and shortcomings and let them drop. But if you do not forgive, neither will your Father in heaven forgive your failings and shortcomings* (Mark 11:25, 26 AMP).

In *Counseling Through Your Bible Handbook,* by June Hunt, an entire chapter is devoted to the subject of forgiveness. Under the title "Forgiveness: The Freedom of Letting Go," Hunt declares that "forgiveness is dismissing a debt, dismissing your demand that others owe you something. Forgiveness is releasing your resentment, releasing your right to hear 'I'm sorry' or the right to get even." She further asserts, "Forgiveness is as much about you as your offender. It removes from you the weight of resentment, freeing you to live a life of joy and peace . . . forgiveness is not letting the guilty off the hook. It is moving the guilty from your hook to God's hook."

HOW DO I ACTUALLY FORGIVE?

June Hunt shares the following strategies to help in forgiving others:

1. Make a list of all the offender's offenses—they are your "rocks" of resentment.
2. Imagine a hook attached to your neck.
3. Imagine a burlap bag filled with those heavy rocks hanging from the hook.
4. Imagine carrying the weight from these burdens everywhere.
5. Ask, "Do I really want to carry all this pain the rest of my life?" (Obviously not!)

6. Now take your offender and the offenses off your emotional hook and put all the pain and this person onto God's hook. The Lord knows how to handle it all, in His time and in His way. "*It is mine to avenge; I will repay*" (Deuteronomy 32:35).

This is a simple strategy to overcome the sin of unforgiveness. It is simple yet so powerful for deliverance. Jesus demonstrated how to forgive when He took our sins while on the cross. He did it to liberate us from accusations, condemnation, judgment, and shame. Try this strategy when an accusing finger is being pointed at you, but you know you are innocent, Try to place yourself in Jesus' situation when He was accused by the religious leaders of His day of blasphemy, or being equal with God. I often think about people who are being accused of some wrongful deed and only the one accused, God and the accuser know the truth. The sad point I want to bring out is how family, friends and acquaintances will judge, condemn, be critical of and agree with the accuser even when they know your character. Many times a person is declared guilty without substantial facts.

I was hired for a position and was told that my orientation would be for ninety days. As the process of orientation went forth, some in leadership came to me and said things that I had not heard from the director. It made me think I was in the wrong place. The one who hired me was out for two weeks; in the meantime I heard different versions of how my schedule would be for the management position. After being employed some approximately twenty-four days someone asked me to go visit patients. I was not prepared to use their computer in the field. I went out and realized that my computer was not fully set up as it should be, so I had issues. I had not been properly trained to understand how to use the computer according to their policy and procedure. Remember, I have only been with the company three weeks. There were different issues that day. All that week I was asked to visit patients around 6:00AM, and come back to the office to take on line courses, train for Clinical Manager and go back out until approximately 6:00PM. I voiced my concerns about being fully prepared to go out to see patients and be in the office all day. I was accused of not wanting to follow directions, refusing to see patients, not following chain of commands, writing a poor order and three other things. The other management person stood in my face and said I had sent a wrong order. I reminded her that I had waited for two days for her to assist me in how to send it, and that it was not me who sent an incomplete order. I was written up for something I did not do. I had to pray for strength to forgive the other manager; it was a struggle for about a week. When I released them to the Lord I received peace; the Lord knew, I knew, and they knew that the complaints were not valid. I actually could not prove it at the time. There are many who are unjustly accused and you know you are innocent. Do not worry but in due season the truth will come forth. If it is not revealed, trust God to work it out in your best interest, for your good. The day I released them I had peace that I had not had for a few days. Your adversary wants to steal your peace.

Forgiving others has been an issue at times for me in the past. During those times I have struggled with forgiveness, I remind myself I will be better, not bitter. Why do women wound other women, intentionally? Sometimes, it could be a root problem that stems from childhood. Parents are supposed to protect their children and when this does not happen, a child can become wounded from simple neglect, or even abuse. I have spoken with women who were sexually abused by male family members and when asked "Did you tell your mother?" answered, "Yes." Some have reported, "My mother said I was lying." Others declared that their mothers ordered, "keep it in the family." One mother even told her daughter that she was at fault for the sexual molestation and was not to say anything about it to anyone.

Some girls or young women may reject a woman who walks in authority or as a "mother figure," because they are reminded of their own mother. There may be some resentment against their own mother who failed to reach out to protect, love, and support . . . at the most vulnerable times in their growth and development stage. Can you imagine the fear, guilt, shame, and betrayal a child must have experienced in not having someone they trust to help them in a time of such dire need?

Wounded people wound others because there is, sometimes, no one they feel they can trust to help heal them of their broken heart. Denial, pretense, deception, and lies are defense mechanisms developed as a result of feeling alone in a situation that did not arise from within. In *Release*, Flora Slosson Wuellner calls this "communal wounding" and offers the following description: "Rigid, embattled walls of separation are the opposite of the radiant healthy borders . . . Nevertheless; the defensive walls grew as a way of survival during our powerlessness. They were a shield for an inner self which was totally vulnerable and which had experienced abuse of trust."

The Lord revealed to me something about trust in September 2010, which I now share with you: When you come out of abuse you enter into a new environment. It is difficult to accept the new environment of peace, freedom, love, and kindness because you have been programmed to tolerate the other. It is like a baby who has been cradled in the mother's womb for nine months; it is warm, comfortable, loving, nurturing, nourishing and secure. Outside of the womb, infants have to depend on someone to know and meet their needs. They are now exposed to foreign surroundings, to an unfamiliar environment. If you are there to tend to that immediate cry or need, the child learns to trust . . . to know that after a while when I cry, someone with warm, cuddly, gentle, loving, nurturing, and nourishing hands will come to my refuge. If someone is not there for the infant to meet their needs mistrust develops. Trust versus mistrust is developed during the infancy stage of growth and development.

Just as the infant has to develop trust in a different environment, so it is with a woman coming out of an abusive situation. The new place for her will have to be a safe, quiet, nurturing, loving and kind environment for a season in order for her to learn how to trust all over again. It does not happen because we speak it; it takes time to recover from abuse; and it takes time to forgive your abuser.

The first time someone displays signs of correction or discipline in love, the wounded individual takes it personally and cries out like an infant. They regress to old memories of abuse and exhibit such emotions as hurt, anger, frustration, strife or low self esteem. The Israelites are a good example: In anguish they cried out to go back to Egypt every time they felt their needs were not going to be met. They even challenged Moses to the point of threatening to kill him if their needs were not met right away. They accused him of bringing them out of Egypt to die in the wilderness. They had been enslaved for over four hundred years and had never experienced autonomy. They suffered from mental, emotional, and physical abuse for so long, they could not enjoy their freedom; they had not learned to trust.

Wounded women do wound other women and this sometimes surfaces as a spirit of jealousy. In my Christian journey

I have seen women oppose other women in leadership just for the sake of doing so . . . respect for women in leadership is not generally given as it is for the men in the same role. The spirit of jealousy—a murdering force—resides within the kingdom of Satan; and whether it is a physical murder or through slander, it is still damaging.

Domestic violence is sometimes motivated by a spirit of jealousy—maybe not in every scenario, as in my case: My former spouse (now deceased) accused me of things I was not guilty of . . . and questioned me about everything I did. He believed in physically abusing a woman if he thought she was lying. He was not born again, and I was in a backslidden state; together we were a mess, trying to survive in our own strength. I had walked away from my former lifestyle as a born-again child of God, suffering many pitfalls as a result of living as a heathen rather than as a [true follower of] Christ.

Those who physically abuse others have a way of inflicting pain on the abused so that it will not be visible to others. My former spouse would hit me in the head when I did not suspect it; and though I fought back, he would prevail. A man is usually stronger than a woman. He smoked marijuana and drank Vodka; and, at times, I was unaware that he was drinking because I could not smell the Vodka. There were times when everything was peaceful . . . then other times when he would become furious with suspicious rage, for no reason. He had spiritual and emotional issues, and so did I.

I was not surrounded by Christian folk during my first marriage; those were years I had left my first love and had settled for satisfying the lust of my flesh. Neither reading the Word of God nor praying was part of my life, even though I attended church. My life was evidenced by an abusive relationship I had settled for, which could have been devastating for both of us.

I finally tired of it all . . . went into another relationship, which was not the right thing to do, for we both were married at the time. It happened over thirty-five years ago, and we both divorced our spouses, which I regretted for years. My regret was not in leaving my first husband but in knowing God was not pleased with me for not seeking His will—so wounded was I that I ended up wounding another woman.

A wounded person thinks only about herself or himself, about getting what he or she wants. The man I am with now is the man I got into a relationship with then; he was kind to me from the beginning and it did not take long for me to trust him. He said that their marriage was on the brink . . . my selfishness said I did not want to be alone. He was my choice—not God's choice for me. We have been married for 30 years, and with both of us coming into the relationship with junk, mess, and 'stuff' it had to be the Lord who delivered us and kept us together over the years.

I eventually had to find forgiveness and peace in the Lord, not in a man. I left the secular church I was in and joined another church. For five years we lived together before getting married in 1981; it was still a few years more before I had peace about the marriage—I felt as if I was out of God's will for a long time. When you are a self-willed person, there are ill-willed consequences to pay. We rededicated ourselves to the Lord in the 1980's and have been faithful to our Christian walk. Our former spouses are both deceased, and have been for over twenty years. I forgave my former husband and was able to lead him to Christ a few months before he died. The last time I visited him in the hospital he was not in a state to recognize me or anyone else due to terminal illness from cancer—probably caused by incessant smoking. I have been grateful to the Lord for allowing me to be the person God used to minister salvation to him, which he received before he passed from this life.

My life began changing as I surrendered daily to the leading of the Holy Spirit. After beginning to study and meditate on the Word of God, I experienced radical life changes: I learned Scriptures and memorized those that were pertinent for my life application. God's Word gave me the strength and fortitude to change. I had no one to counsel me but the Holy Spirit; He led me to the Scriptures to help me in my time of need. I listened to God's Word during worship at our church, developed a strong prayer life, and learned to praise and worship the Lord.

During my more than twenty-two year as a minister, I have gleaned from my pastors, from watching Christian television, specifically Trinity Broadcasting Network (TBN), and others. My initial journey as a minister learning was enhanced by leaders such as my pastor, Dr. Fred Price, Pastor Benny Hinn, Brother Kenneth Hagin, Sr., Minister Marilyn Hickey, and others. Later on, God brought other anointed spiritual leaders into my life; two very special ones were instrumental in assisting us to plant the first church: Elder William (Bill) Frazier (currently residing in Atlanta with his spouse Barbara) and his mother Sister Maxine Frazier (now deceased). They were true prayer warriors, and Elder Bill was powerful in teaching God's Word; they assisted us in edifying and equipping God's people. It is important to have others to pour into your life.

It is important to have wise counselors or coaches. Initially I did not have counselors afforded to me; thus, my road to recovery was much longer. Because of shame and guilt, I did not want to share my story with a counselor or a pastor—and that is a trick of the devil! The Message Bible states, "*Make this your common practice, confess your sins to each other and pray for each other so that you can live together whole and healed. The prayer of a person living right with God is something powerful to be reckoned with*" (James 5:16).

James discusses the reason for fights and wars that originate within us, for it is important to get an understanding of why these behaviors manifest:

> *What leads to strife (discord and feuds) and how do conflicts (quarrels and fightings) originate among you? Do they not arise from your sensual desires that are ever warring in your bodily members? You are jealous and covet [what others have] and your desires go unfulfilled; [so] you become murderers. [To hate is to murder as far as your hearts are concerned.] You burn with envy and anger and are not able to obtain [the gratification, the contentment, and the happiness that you seek], so you fight and war. You do not have, because you do not ask* (James 4:1, 2 AMP).

James ascertains why so much strife and discord exists among God's people, ungodly attributes one expects to see from those who do not have a relationship with the Lord, not from those who profess to know Christ:

> *[Or] you do ask [God for them] and yet fail to receive, because you ask with wrong purpose and evil, selfish motives. Your intention is [when you get what you desire] to spend it in sensual pleasures. You [are like] unfaithful wives [having illicit love affairs with*

> *the world and breaking your marriage vow to God]! Do you know that being the world's friend is being God's enemy? So whoever chooses to be a friend of the world takes his stand as an enemy of God* (James 4:3, 4 AMP).

There are several cases in the Hebrew Bible of women wounding other women due to jealousy. This stems from the days when Lucifer the archangel of worship had full dominion on the earth. His rulership under God happened during the pre-Adamite universe. He became jealous of God and purposed in his heart to dethrone Him, instead Lucifer was cast out of heaven, and became our adversary, Satan.

> *How art thou fallen from heaven, O Lucifer, son of the morning! How art thou cut down to the ground, which didst weaken the nations! For thou hadst said in thine heart, I will ascend into heaven, I will exalt my throne above the stars of God. I will sit also upon the mount of the congregation, in the sides of the north. I will ascend above the heights of the clouds; I will be like the most High. Yet thou shalt be brought down to hell, to the sides of the pit.* Isaiah 14: 12-15.

Lucifer was a created angel, an anointed cherub. Angels are cherubs not human beings. God made Him perfect in all of his ways, until iniquity (lawlessness) was found in his heart. God set this cherub over the first earth to protect it, overshadow it, and to rule it. He became defiled because of his beauty, therefore arrogance and pride became a stronghold for Lucifer. After so long, and we do not know how long he became jealous of God and decided according to Isaiah that he would dethrone Him. Ezekiel 28: 11-19 teaches about his beauty, his role, and how slander against God caused him to lose his place in the Kingdom of God. The dethroned cherub is now our adversary and he tries to defeat us because of the victory Christ won for us on the cross and through his Resurrection.

Jealousy had been a stronghold before the foundations of the earth, as we have previously read. It is not a stronghold that women only are plagued with, but it a demonic force that attacks men and children as well. I want to emphasize women for the purpose of the focus for this Chapter. I want to discuss women who were put in a position to be jealous and also to overcome it. In the Hebrew Bible during Abraham's time on earth, men were allowed to practice polygamy; they were allowed two or more wives for the purpose of procreation. Even though it was customary in Jewish culture, wives of the same husband were bound to be resentful and jealous of each other.

The story of Abram and Sarai is proof that the other woman did cause a problem for the marriage. Sarai was elderly and well beyond the child-bearing age—barren. She instructed her spouse Abram to lie with her maid Hagar, so that a child would be born to that union. Abram listened to Sarai and took Hagar as his second wife. The civil laws stated that children born from a master and a slave girl would belong to the master. "*… he had intercourse with Hagar, and she became pregnant; and when she saw that she was with child, she looked with contempt upon her mistress and despised her*" (Genesis 16:4 AMP).

Webster defines *contempt* as "disdain, scorn hatred, and disrespect." The word *despised* means disdain (to regard as beneath one's dignity), scorn, disrespect, or hatred." You can see then how the woman under authority came to despise or abhor the woman in authority. To be barren in the Jewish culture was not an accepted practice; the Egyptian slave girl knew it and tried to use it to her advantage.

Hagar and Sarai more than likely were both wounded. Sarai's wounded state came out of being barren for seventy-five years. The slave girl Hagar looked upon Sarai with scorn and hatred after she became pregnant by Sarai's husband Abram. When Sarai decided Hagar should have a child by Abram, Hagar had no choice in the decision making; she was given over to an older man to be sexually intimate with him, whether she agreed or not. That was the custom during that era. Nevertheless, all rights were essentially denied Hagar as a bonds woman; she was subjected to the demands of another person who had power over her. Hagar became haughty after she conceived; she forgot that she was still a slave with no rights and that Abram only yielded to Sarai's request because he knew she desired a child. Not being able to make a decision about your personal life and the child to be born must have been depressing for Hagar.

Sarai suffered shame and disgrace as a result of her barrenness. Then she had to endure mockery from her bond maid once conception took place with Sarai's husband. Can you imagine the hurt Sarai must have felt? She gave Hagar to Abram for the purpose of procreation and Hagar rejected Sarai after conception occurred. What would you have done? I can imagine Sarai being sorry a thousand times over for trying to assist God in easing her pain and suffering, trying to also help Abram to fulfill God's promise to him. Here is a lesson for all to learn from: God does not need our help in fulfilling the promises He had made to us. All we need to do is trust and wait on Him.

In a previous chapter, the story of Hannah is discussed in order to see how this woman—also barren—longed for a child. Hannah, too, was belittled, mocked, scorned, laughed at and discouraged by the second wife, Peninnah. Peninnah was fruitful in bearing children for Elkanah (Hannah's husband) and was jealous of Hannah, because Elkanah loved Hannah more than he did her. Peninnah was wounded, therefore leading to the theory, "wounded people do wound others."

In the case of Jacob, Leah, and Rachel, the scenario was similar, but in a sense it was worse, because these two women were sisters—married to the same man. Leah could have children but Rachel could not conceive. Jacob loved Rachel more than he did Leah and was tricked into marrying Leah by their father. On the wedding night, their father Laban switched the sisters—Rachel for Leah. Only after consummation (sexual intercourse) of the vows did Jacob realize he had married the wrong sister! (Leah was wearing a veil and this is why Jacob did not discover who she was initially.) Surely, none of us could imagine the hurt from such deception.

> *And Jacob served seven years for Rachel, and they seemed to him but a few days because of the love he had for her. Finally, Jacob said to Laban, Give me my wife, for my time is completed, so that I may take her to me. And Laban gathered together all the men of the place and made a feast. But when night came he took Leah his daughter and brought her to Jacob, who had intercourse with her* (Genesis 29:20-23, 25 Msg).

Can you see the trickery and deception in this narrative? Remember Jacob and his mother Rebekah deceived Isaac, his father. Isaac was elderly and his eyesight was poor, so Jacob's mother with his agreement schemed for

Jacob to be blessed by Isaac rather than the eldest son, Esau. Jacob stole his brother's birthright according to Genesis 27. He was a deceiver until God changed his name to Israel. Remember, whatever you do to others will be done to you. Jacob engaged in deception with his mother and his mother's brother deceived him. It looks like a generational curse in the family that needed to be broken.

> *But in the morning Jacob saw his wife and behold it was Leah! And he said to Laban, 'What is this you have done to me? Did I not work for you [all those seven years] for Rachel? Why then have you deceived and cheated and thrown me down like this?'* (Genesis 29:25, Msg).

Laban did eventually give Rachel to Jacob in marriage; he had to work seven additional years to fulfill his vow to Laban in order to marry her. Jacob loved Rachel. Leah realized that Rachel was loved more by Jacob so she was always seeking ways to manipulate him into loving her. Jacob's marriage to Leah was set up by her dad—Jacob had no plans to marry her. Laban wanted the first daughter married before the second daughter—according to Jewish custom. It all had to be painful for the wives, who were sisters, as well as for Jacob.

When Rachel saw that she bore Jacob no children, she envied her sister, and said to Jacob, Give me children, or else I will die! And Jacob became angry with Rachel and he said, Am I in God's stead, Who has denied you children? (Genesis 30:1, 2 AMP). She probably spoke a curse over herself, because immediately after she had her second child, Rachel died. We must ask the Lord to put a guard over our mouth so that we do not say things that can later be a snare to us: "*You are snared with the words of your lips; you are caught by the speech of your mouth*" (Proverbs 6:2 AMP).

The women began to give their maids to Jacob, so that children would be born through their union with their husband. Rachel had been married to Jacob for some years before she conceived:

> *Then God remembered Rachel and answered her pleading and made it possible for her to have children. And [now for the first time] she became pregnant and bore a son; and she said, God has taken away my reproach, disgrace, and humiliation* (Genesis 30:22, 23 AMP).

You can visualize the pain, suffering, and slander Rachel must have endured for not being able to conceive, and the contention that was on-going between the two sisters in sharing the same man. Truly, this story also supports the theory that "wounded women wound other women."

David A. Seamands shares in his book, *Healing for Damaged Emotions,* that Satan uses psychological tactics to try and wear down God's people: "Satan's greatest psychological weapon is a gut-level feeling of inferiority, inadequacy, and low self-worth. This feeling shackles many Christians, in spite of wonderful experiences and in spite of their faith and knowledge of God's Word. Although they understand their position as sons and daughters of God, they are tied up in knots, bound by a terrible feeling of inferiority, and chained to a deep sense of worthlessness"

Seamands posits, "There are four ways that Satan uses this deadliest of all of his emotional and psychological weapons, to bring defeat and failure into your life:

1. Low self-esteem paralyzes your potential.
2. Low self-esteem destroys your dreams.
3. Low self-esteem ruins your relationship.
4. Low self-esteem sabotages your Christian service.

I agree with him, for, at times, I have felt inadequate . . . not worthy to lead God's people. Whenever there was an exodus from the church during my pastorate, I was left feeling as if I had failed in some area as a pastor. It is not always easy to remain calm when someone who sat under your ministry leaves out and tries to discredit you for helping them. I have seen it happen so many times; and it has usually been women in the ministry who were overlooked by previous leaders, or someone coveting a gift God had not set them in. Usually wounded when they arrive, their wounds are superficially covered. They confess primarily of being hurt by their former church and pastor(s), believing they were overlooked or not affirmed. The real issue is not the hurt received from the former church, which may have stirred up memories, thoughts, and emotions; it more than likely stems from rejection felt even earlier in their past.

Oftentimes, women who are called into the Lord's ministry are not willing to discuss the possibility of their having left their former ministry in error. They may have an aught against their former pastor(s), especially if there is a female co-pastor. Of course, this may also apply to men. As pastors we fail many times to help them receive their deliverance and healing by failing to find out why they left. We are so glad to take in people as members that we forget many come in broken, bruised, battered, and disappointed with the church and spiritual leaders. We do God, the church, and the individual(s) a disservice when we do not take the time to assess and evaluate their purpose for leaving their previous church.

In talking with them initially you will discern whether they indeed are wounded. The members may not discern, but, as a pastor, you will be able to. If so, it is important that they sit until healed internally—otherwise, someone will be hurt from their hemorrhaging, sarcasm, jealousy, competition, envy, strife, division, and slander. Such hurt may be rooted in childhood abuse, marital abuse, generational curses, neglect, and misuse by those whom they trusted; nevertheless, they have been sent to be delivered and healed. Some will leave prematurely when all is revealed.

Wounded women who wound other women present a genuine issue that needs to be addressed in our churches. There is so much envy and competition among women; and this should not be. Women who are in Christ are powerful and a force to be reckoned with.

Chuck D. Pierce, in *The Future War of the Church,* states, "Many women struggle to understand all they are in Christ. They have been told over and over again, 'Here's your role.' The enemy has used this (old) religious spirit to steal women's hope and confine them to a place the Lord never intended." Women uniting together could bring about a transition in this earth that will produce order to much of the chaos. They give birth; they are warriors, worshippers, nurturers, healers, comforters; God knows how He created them and what He has created them to do. Anointed women are powerful in the prayer room as intercessors:

> *Thus says the Lord of hosts, Consider and call for the mourning women to come, send for the skillful women to come. Let them make haste and raise a wailing over us, that our eyes may run down with tears and our eyelids gush with water . . . Yet hear the Word of the Lord, O you women, and let your ears*

> *receive the word of His mouth; teach your daughters a lament (how to mourn) and each one [teach] her neighbor a dirge* (Jeremiah 9:17,18, 20 AMP).

Jeremiah the prophet was speaking from the mouth of God: "*For death has come up into our windows, it has entered into our palaces, cutting off the children from outdoors and the young men from the streets*" (Jeremiah 9:21 AMP).

The destruction of our land and scattering of our children is happening today as it did during Jeremiah's day. Today, we hear of children being kidnapped and later found to be in forced sex slavery, or dead. We hear about murders constantly occurring on the streets in our communities. The unemployment rate is continuing to escalate, people are losing their homes, and marriages are failing daily. The traditional family is shifting because of differences in sexual preferences. Domestic violence is on the increase; drug infestation has destroyed neighborhoods, and the census in the jails and prisons grow larger daily.

In Jeremiah's day God scattered His people because of their rebellion and disobedience to Him. God allowed an unrighteous nation to capture them, destroy their city, take their goods, and remove them to a foreign land. This happened because they continued to go after false gods and false worship. The Israelites worshipped foreign idols without reverence to the Holy God, Creator of heaven and earth.

We need the mourning women to come together. We must send for the skillful women who know how to wail over our land and God's people, so that reconciliation and restoration will happen supernaturally. As we have seen in this chapter, women operating in strife, contention, jealousy, competition, envy, and unforgiveness cannot fulfill their God-given purpose. Too much time is wasted in trying to please the flesh; but through our travailing in prayer, we can birth some things in the spirit and see them manifested—that all will come into the knowledge of Christ and His redeeming power.

Satan hates women because we bring forth the seed. In the Garden of Eden after the fall of Adam and Eve, God spoke to the serpent, saying, "*And I will put enmity between you and the woman, and between your offspring and her Offspring. He will bruise and tread your head underfoot, and you will lie in wait and bruise His heel*" (Genesis 3:15 AMP).

God put hostility between the serpent and the woman in the Garden of Eden after Adam and Eve fell into disobedience. Satan, who appeared to the woman in the form of a serpent, was trying to discredit God and make them doubt God's Word. He failed and they fell; but God did not.

Pierce further states, ". . . Satan hates women with great wrath. One way you can always determine the level of the antichrist spirit and his operation is how you see women being treated in a region. Similarly, how you see women being treated in the church displays the level of the freedom of God in that region. The two are in direct correlation with each other."

We have an adversary; so it is important that we join forces together and take authority over everything that would try to hinder and stop us as we move forward. The Book of James discusses the necessity of having genuine faith to produce results in good works: "*Is anyone among you afflicted (ill-treated, suffering evil)? He (she) should pray. Is anyone glad at heart? He (she) should sing praise to God*" (James 5:13). This is why we cannot be at each other's throat in ministry, for as women we must fulfill our God-given purpose for being on this earth. Time is short in comparison to eternity; it is not to be wasted engaging in unproductive, idle, aimless, and unnecessary foolishness.

There was an internet article from Joyce Meyer's Magazine titled "Welcoming Inner Healing," written by Paul Meier, M.D. and Esly Regina Carvalho, M.S. LPC. The article states, "One thing that God has been speaking to us about in the last few years is that without inner healing—the healing of the soul—people do not get to the level of holiness that God has called His church to live. It is clear in the Word that God desires to raise up godly offspring and He wants a holy church. As Christian counselors we often ask ourselves, "Why doesn't this happen more frequently in the church?"

The article goes on to state, "Both of us constantly see people who want to live healthier lives. They often come to us in horrific emotional pain as a result of disappointments, rejections and even personal failures—spiritual and otherwise. We encourage them with the good news that they can grow healthier mentally and emotionally with God's help. But first they will need to recognize and deal with some things that often get in the way of experiencing God's best."

Dr. Meier and Esly Carvalho posed the following question about healing, and offered some steps toward getting help:

CAN WE LEARN TO HEAL AND BE HOLY?

1. **Take It To Jesus.** Ask Him to heal the broken pieces of your fragmented life that only He can heal, making you a healthy, whole person again. I [Esly] love the words of Malachi 4:2 NIV: '*But for you who revere my name, the sun of righteousness will rise with healing in its wings . . . .* ' Like a little chick that cuddles up to the warm heart of its mother, we are also called to come near the breast of God and listen to His heartbeat. It's there that the Lord tenderly speaks to us with words of healing and binds up our bruised lives.

2. **Seek the Truth About Yourself.** Exercise courage: Ask God to give you a spirit of wisdom and revelation so that you can see any sin that hinders you. David prayed in Psalm 139 and asked God to shine His searchlight in his soul and reveal his secret sins and wounds. You too can pray for truth to be revealed, knowing that only the truth will set you free from the continual bondage of depression and misery.

3. **Meditate on Scripture.** Ask God to lead you to passages that will give you insights into your unconscious thoughts, feelings and motives. Hebrews 4:12 tells us that the Word of God is sharp, like a two-edged sword, revealing our innermost thoughts and motives.

4. **Fellowship with People.** As iron sharpens iron, we need trustworthy friends to be honest with us about what they see in us that may need a little tuning up. James 5:16 promises that as we confess our sins to one another, we will be healed.

5. **Seek Professional Help.** Believe it or not, when you go see a professional Christian counselor once a week or more for your emotional pain, they are actually discipling you. Christian counselors are trained to dig up root causes of the problems people face and reveal them to their clients in love.

6. **Obey What You Know.** For inner healing to occur, we need to know the truth to uncover the root of our problems. But once we discover the truth, we must walk in obedience to it in order to be set free. Although obedience itself does not heal directly, it does put us in that place of protection where healing can occur. God's will for our lives is good, perfect and pleasing. For those who doubt this, I [Esly] tell them to try the alternative—disobedience. It won't take them long to get a quick lesson on how painful it is to live outside the will of God.

7. **God Works Healing In Us As Long As We Remain In Obedience.** As we walk in His ways our souls are healed and we develop holiness; we also stop complicating our lives with the consequences of additional sin. In His grace and mercy God speaks tenderly to our hearts and develops the character of Jesus in us. And it is through His death, burial and resurrection that we are set free from sin and able to enjoy restored fellowship near the Father.

Meier and Carvalho continue by saying, "Romans 8:29 tells us that God's goal for our lives is to make us more and more like Jesus—in our thoughts, feelings, motives, and actions. This will take willingness and effort on our part, coupled with the abiding power of the Holy Spirit to strengthen us along the way. "*And don't forget that . . . in an abundance of counselors there is victory and safety"* (Proverbs 24:6). So be open and humble enough to ask specialists in various fields for help. And, most importantly, ask the Holy Spirit to guide you to the right help at the right time to arrive at the right conclusions."

Meier and Carvalho remind us that "we are all born with imperfections and defects . . God can heal anything, but He often uses our weaknesses to develop our trust and reliance upon Him, as well as our character. The need for medication is not a sign of failure or a lack of faith, as some have been taught . . . There are some individuals who have chemical imbalances in their brain. Thankfully, we now know that medication can correct this disorder and many others in a number of people."

7

SIGNS, WONDERS, AND MIRACLES CONCERNING HEALING

This concluding chapter focuses on how God heals using God's principles that involve nothing but divine intervention. We say 'God heals, but . . .?' I want you to know that God does heal in the 21st century without interventions from modern technology or pharmaceutical products. At one point in Jesus' ministry, He said, "*. . . If you can believe, all things are possible to him* (her) *(who believes)*" (Mark 9:23 NKJV).

Is there anything too hard for God? The answer is 'No.' We believe Him for homes, cars, and other material things, why not believe Him for our healing—whether it is physical, spiritual, emotional, or mental. We can absolutely recover all when we put our faith in the Word of God, including finances. Everything that pertains to life and godliness has been given unto us; it is a Kingdom of God principle:

> *[After all] the kingdom of God is not a matter of [getting the] food and drink [one likes], but instead it is righteousness (that state which makes a person acceptable to God) and [heart] peace and joy in the Holy Spirit. He who serves Christ in this way is acceptable and pleasing to God and is approved by men. So let us definitely aim for and eagerly pursue what makes for harmony and for mutual upbuilding (edification and development) of one another* (Romans 14:17-19 AMP).

An elder, at one time a member of my church before I moved to Atlanta in 2003, reminded me of the time she called me to pray for her brother. It was a few years ago, maybe 2002, when the physician announced that her brother was dead. After we prayed God revived him supernaturally. What an awesome God we are in covenant with! Her brother eventually passed on, but God did allow him to live after having been pronounced dead. I had forgotten about God raising him up because at the time we were praying for so many people. Later, I recalled him being in the Hospice Unit of the hospital; that he had actually been pronounced dead; that we prayed for him in the room, and God did raise him up!

We operate under the anointing of the Holy Spirit to help restore health to those who are sick, diseased, or infirmed. It is one way to promote mutual edification and development of one another. The anointing is the power of the Holy Spirit, or divine enablement which we are graced to operate in to set the captives free. No one wants to be held captive if there is a way out. We as believers in Christ must demonstrate to others the greater works that Jesus discussed with His disciples. As men and women of God, when we teach and preach the principles of God's Kingdom, manifestations of His presence and power are evident with tangible results: The sick are healed, the demonized are delivered, and the wounded are made whole. Those in long periods of mourning receive a release from the spirit of heaviness and begin to be joyful.

We need to change the atmosphere around us by declaring the Word of God concerning divine healing. *Faith Healing Ministry: A Christian Education Model for Clergy and Laity* is the title of my dissertation. In it I contend that the ministry of healing should be in all Christian ministries. Some may ask, "Why is it necessary?" It is necessary so that the body may be healed and made whole. There has even been a paradigm shift in how some physicians and scientists accept the importance of their patients in relation to faith and prayer. They have seen the effects of prayer and faith in some of their patients who practice their beliefs and values. There is documented proof that these patients have favorable outcomes in comparison to the patients who do not practice faith and belief in God. In 1982-83, a study was done in San Francisco General Medical Coronary Care Unit, which demonstrated that hospitalized heart patients had fewer medical complications when prayed for than when not. The evidence was published in the Southern Medical Journal:

> Physicians and scientists have observed the importance of prayer and faith in the recovery of their patients, and some are encouraging their patients in their religious practices. The Christian church at one time understood their role in healing, it was the center for healing. Clergy has rescinded in their role as spiritual healers and relegated healing for the body of Christ to modern medicine and technology. From the research and participation in the program it suggests to the author that Christian education is

needed to re- trieve the ministry of faith healing. The ultimate goal is to take the heal- ing message to the world to draw others to know the love of God for humanity.

There was a time the physicians and clergy (ordained ministers) worked as a team. "The portrait of Medicus and Clericus, physicians and clergy, as partners in healing is a common one throughout the evangelical tradition. It was symbolized for them in two biblical figures, the missionaries Luke and Paul; the one a beloved physician whose care was for the body, the other a spiritual leader whose care was for the soul. The two together provided evangelicals with a holistic model of Jesus' ministry of teaching, preaching, and healing as described in Matthew."

The gospels Matthew, Mark, Luke, and John describe the ministry of Jesus during his mission of earth. All of it could not be recorded in the biblical record, it was so vast. The evangelicals and the physicians modeled after the ministry of Jesus according to the Book of Matthew. Healing wounded people is one way God relates to the world to demonstrate His love and providence to humankind.

Evangelical is "a term used in Europe for Protestant. In America it has come to refer to one who stresses the need for a personal relationship with God in Jesus Christ by faith. Some who claim the term seek to define it further in terms of theological beliefs about particular issues," (McKim, 96)

In researching my dissertation I discovered the root cause of this division between physicians and clergy working together to heal. Modernity is "a term used to designate the post –Enlightenment period in Europe and North America in which people turned to a scientific culture and its promises in order to fill a void left by a decline in religion. The values of the secular culture and rejection of religious authority are primary, as well as a belief in knowledge as certain, objective, and good," (McKim, 176). This definition helps in making you aware of the paradigm shift that took place during the Modern Era.

> Modern science and the professionalism of modern life labored to separate Medicus and Clericus until evangelicalism's high model of partnership became a subdominant part of its tradition. Euphoric over the fact that they could really heal, physicians for much of the twentieth century decided to go at it alone in the healing enterprise. The division between physicians and clergy (ministers) widened due to the church becoming euphoric over modern medicine's miracles and unsure about its own offerings to the healing enterprise . . . 'science brought medicine almost to the border of the miraculous,' in the words of one evangelical, the pastoral function of the church upheld a safe, respectful distance from medical and healing matters. Religion joined the rest of the culture in cheering on medical technology as it, in Ivan Illich's words, 'began to reclai*m* the right to perform miracles'. . . the two professions became separated, in *Healing and Medicine in the Evangelical Tradition: Neither by Might nor Power,* by Leonard I. Sweet.(p. 141).

Some theological doctrines have been effective in the cessation of the gifts of the Spirit operating within the body of Christ. In trying to understand God in how He relates to us as human beings, we have a tendency to miss some pertinent revelation in how He deals with humanity. Healing is one of the nine supernatural gifts of the Spirit:

> *But to each one is given the manifestation of the [Holy] Spirit, [the evidence, the spiritual illumination of the Spirit] for good and profit. To one is given in and through the [Holy] Spirit [the power to speak] a message of wisdom, and to another [the power to express] a word of knowledge and understanding according to the same [Holy] Spirit; To another [wonder-working] faith by the same Holy Spirit; to another the extraordinary powers of healing by the one Spirit; To another the working of miracles, to another prophetic insight (the gift of interpreting the divine will and purpose); to another the ability to discern and distinguish between the[utterances of true] spirits [and false ones], to another various kinds of [unknown] tongues, to another the ability to interpret [such] tongues. All these [gifts, achievements, abilities] are inspired and brought to pass by one and the same [Holy] Spirit, Who apportions to each person individually [exactly] as He chooses (1Corinthians 12:7-11 AMP).*

In Benjamin B. Warfield's classic, *Counterfeit Miracles,* he was adamant about his theory concerning the cessation of miracles. He joined in with Martin Luther, John Calvin, and John Wesley in their theological views. All three argues in one form or another that miracles were, in Calvin's words, 'a temporary gift,' although Wesley pushed God's withdrawal of miracles well into the third century and then only because of the 'church's decay of faith.' All the reformers contended that God allowed the spoken Word to pre-empt the healing gifts. Warfield contended that 'after the apostolic age miracles ceased,' because God's Word was demonstrated with signs and wonders to be proof of the supernatural. Miracles were only to launch the faith and manifest Christ's deity.

We have a better understanding of why the ministry of healing is an almost lost ministry in most denominations or churches. The body of Christ has been influenced by church reformers and the Modern Era.

Christ suffered so that believers in Him would not have to suffer with the same issues. As parents we have pioneered and established businesses, ministries, and some successful inventions so that our children can reap the benefits of our labor. If they heed to how the Holy Spirit is guiding them, they will reap a great harvest and will not have the struggles we experienced. The ground has already been plowed; the forerunners broke up the fallow ground. God has used some of us as parents to break up fallow ground for our seeds. It is the same way with the mistakes we have made as parents; we try to spare our children so that they will not have to experience the same mistakes. We warn them of the pitfalls, but it is up to them to listen and change their course of action.

Jesus has gone before us to prepare the way—to rid us of all curses so that we may walk in the liberty He sacrificed His life for us to have. Jesus was beaten with many stripes before His crucifixion and those stripes represented Him being wounded so that we could be healed. They represent major sicknesses and diseases. Jesus bore them for us. Why then should we bear the same curses? It is time to be free. We must recognize, acknowledge, and appreciate what Jesus has done for us at Calvary! We cannot allow His suffering to be in vain. Jesus' death on the cross was a three-fold mission: (1) He was wounded with stripes so that we might be healed; (2) He bore our sins so that we might be liberated without sin having any more dominion over us as believers; and (3) We are also saved from eternal destruction. What a mighty God we serve!

David blessed the Lord for His mercies and admonishes all believers to praise the Lord for what He has done:

> *Bless the LORD, O my soul: and all that is within me, bless His holy name. Bless the LORD, O my soul, and forget not all his benefits: who forgiveth all thine iniquities; who healeth all thy diseases; who redeemeth thy life from destruction; who crowneth thee with loving kindness and tender mercies; who satisfieth thy mouth with good things; so that thy youth is renewed like the eagle's* (Psalms 103:1-5).

My desire is to retrieve the ministry of faith healing or divine healing for the Christian church. It is a ministry not utilized in most churches, but much needed! The ministry of healing is as relevant for today as it has been in the past. I have observed the ministry of [Pastor] Benny Hinn for eighteen years. I have also done some study on the healing ministries of Smiths Wigglesworth, Kathryn Kuhlman, Francis MacNutt, John G. Lake and others. It is my belief that the Lord is pleased with those who have continued to adhere to the Kingdom of God practices, because it benefits the body of Christ.

Healing miracles also point to Jesus. Oftentimes some are drawn to Him because of the blessing that has been poured out on them, which is deemed to be a miracle from God. My study of the ministry of healing began over eighteen years ago after having seen miracles occurring in our ministry for approximately three years. In me developed a burning desire to know more about the supernatural power of God, as it relates to healing. As a child, I saw how God healed some of my family when hands were laid on them, coupled with prayer. I am grateful to the Church of God in Christ (COGIC) and our spiritual leaders who practiced the laying on of hands, with prayer for the sick, diseased, and infirmed. I gleaned from them; it [the gift] was lying dormant in me all of those years.

After acknowledging my call into the ministry in 1988, I fasted from secular television for thirteen years to spend time in God's Word; I believed it and put it into practice. Then a door was opened for me in December 1989, at the Wayside Christian Mission in Louisville, Kentucky to begin weekly Bible study in that Christian homeless shelter. There we taught the Word of God and prayed for folk for over nine years.

December 1990 was the first time I had prayed for someone in a coma; and I witnessed God bring them out of it. It was actually two people whom God healed from a cerebral hemorrhage. During that time my pastor, Bernard Barnes said to me, "I believe God is moving you into the ministry of healing." I began praying for folk between 1990-1992 while on duty as a registered nurse; and I could see God touching lives. Although I began working there in the hospital in 1978, those first few years I was in no position to pray for anyone because I needed deliverance.

It boosted my faith to pray for people everywhere I was allowed to minister. I also included prayer as an intricate part of my nursing profession. I believed God would transform those that I prayed for and do whatever was necessary to make them whole. God allowed us to personally evangelize in drug infested communities, a homeless mission, and in one of the largest prisons in our state. At the Kentucky State Reformatory, many people were delivered and set free; in fact, the guys packed the chapel when Faith Dominion was on the campus.

In 1994 our ministry team went to the Kentucky State Reformatory (KSR) for the first time and witnessed an awesome move of God: We prayed for an inmate there who could not talk; he got baptized with the Holy Ghost and began to speak in tongues, and to also talk naturally. Another person was paralyzed and confined to a wheelchair as a result of trying to escape some years before; he had been sentenced to spend seventy-five years in prison. We were told that he was released shortly after we prayed for him. God is great and greatly to be praised!

Our church was allowed to minister there only three times a year because of the number of other ministries involved with the prison ministry. After moving to Atlanta, I asked my son to oversee the prison ministry, which he did. On returning to Louisville to visit in 2006, I again had the opportunity to be involved in the prison ministry outreach at KSR. We always gave an altar call and men would come for salvation, deliverance, healing, relationship restoration, and various other reasons, We always asked for those to come forth that needed salvation and to be healed, and we would pray for them.

We saw numerous miracles while being involved in this prison ministry. I did not know until 2009 that three years previously I had prayed with a man who was diagnosed with Hepatitis C. He got my attention and reminded me that he had been healed since he was prayed for three years before. There is absolutely nothing God cannot do! Our involvement continued with the prison ministry at KSR until December 2009. With the increase in population at KSR they currently have two chaplains providing Sunday chapel worship for those incarcerated. The doors closed to all ministries providing chapel worship for the men on Sunday. Our ministry had been scheduled for Sunday worship so we do not have the opportunity to participate at the present time.

Sometimes, we need to give credit where credit is due. I heard about the Benny Hinn Ministry in 1992 after returning from Germany. Those who attended the crusade while I was away were so overjoyed by the move of the Holy Spirit that it touched my heart. Someone informed me of Hinn's book, *Good Morning, Holy Spirit,* which I then read. I was not the same after that experience; for three days I was high in the Spirit! I attended his next crusade which was held in Indianapolis, Indiana. I went there searching—knowing God had something more for me to do and desiring to find out what it was. From the moment I entered the stadium I knew what God had called me to do: He had called me to seek His face and to establish a ministry for the sick, diseased, and infirmed in order that they would receive deliverance and healing.

I began to go to crusades approximately twice a year in such places, Chicago, Illinois; St. Louis, Missouri; Cincinnati, Ohio; Columbus, Ohio; Indianapolis, Indiana; Atlanta, Georgia; Nashville, Tennessee, and Louisville, Kentucky. As often as I could, I always took other people with me and, as their pastor, provided transportation for those wanting to attend. Our church was very healthy; we did not have a sick list or people in the hospital. I was a pastor there for twelve years and only one person died during my tenure; and she was not ill. To God be the glory.

Spirit-led worship filled the atmosphere at the crusades during their choir rehearsals; people were receiving their healing before the 7 P M meeting began. The atmosphere was charged with the electrifying power of the Holy Spirit. Worship filled the atmosphere and the Word of God was taught and preached to build faith in the people. I had never experienced anything like it before; I was amazed and at the same time thrust into a dimension of God's glory that I had never before encountered—it was awesome! I fell under the power of God while standing at the top row of seats in the stadium. The things I encountered gave me more of a hunger for Jesus and a deeper desire to pursue His call on my life. It changed my life and my ministry's perspective.

My son Shawn had been in a near-fatal accident and was hospitalized for three months. He was in a car chase with police pursuing him when he hit a parked van and a utility pole. Seven weeks before, he had robbed a store and shot a clerk, but no one knew it was him. He became one of 35 suspects after suffering his accident; he confessed the second day after the crash. I suppose he thought he was going to die; and he died, several times— but God kept reviving him. He was a wayward child at 19 years of age . . . before the accident had moved to New York where he got involved in gangs and drugs. I was praying, fasting, and seeking the Lord for his salvation.

One day he called me from New York and said, without asking me how I was doing, "Mama, quit praying for me." I replied, "I am not going to quit praying for you boy." He was trying to sign a contract with some R & B artist in New York, but it was difficult. The day Shawn called me from New York; the adversary spoke into his ear. "The reason you are not getting the record deal is because someone is praying for you." He knew it was his mother.

He had major surgeries after the accident and was paralyzed from the chest down. In July of 1993, I came out of a courtroom broken, fell into a chair outside the door and cried—my son had been put under a $250,000.00 cash bond, and he could not even sit up in a chair. The Spirit spoke to me and said, "Go to the Benny Hinn Crusade." I knew it was in Chicago but had no plans to attend due to Shawn's court date and my work schedule for that day. At that moment, I requested time off from my employer—explaining what God had spoken. I left at 2 PM and arrived on the grounds of the Rosemont Coliseum at 6:55 PM, five minutes before the start of the crusade.

I ran through the facility crying along with the young lady who was with me, Shawn's friend Shaunta. We ran down some steps and explained to the usher why we were there, and he said, "Lady, take my seat." Shaunta was allowed to sit on the steps adjacent to me. Hot tears ran down my cheeks for three and one-half hours. It did not change my situation but I received an inner healing during the worship. I left the crusade—with an inner knowing that God had moved supernaturally in my behalf..

On the inside I had felt like a total wreck; but I maintained my composure because of being a pastor. I had felt so broken from all the circumstances involving my son. I had to dress to impress—had to cover—so no one would discover how wounded I was. I had to preach on Sundays and teach on Thursdays as if I had it all together. If it had not been for the Lord on my side, I never would have made it! Going to the crusade helped me; the anointing of the Holy Spirit was so thick in the place that I was totally saturated with His presence. Miracles were happening all around me! Emotional healing was happening in me! I was broken and in turmoil when I arrived but when I left, I had peace and confidence that God was in control and that it was working out for our good.

I took a pair of Shawn's pants to the crusade. Before it was over, I was able to give those pants to Pastor Dave

Palmquist and Suzanne Hinn for Pastor Benny to pray over. He did . . . and they brought them back to me. I could not give those pants to Shawn for almost a year, but it was my act of faith in God that caused my son to be healed from multiple wounds and surgeries. One-half of his stomach was removed, his spleen, and his stomach nerves. Rods were put in his back and he could not sit up for over a year without a body cast. Development of *endocarditis*, an infection around his heart, forced Shawn to be on intravenous medication for months. He repented of his sins and *gave his heart* to the Lord Jesus. He began to study and meditate upon the Word of God which gave him strength to endure. Shawn was incarcerated for over six years after giving his heart to Jesus and led other inmates to Christ, or either encouraged them in their Christian walk. We kept visiting him, sharing the Word of God with him, and praying for his full recovery.

I believe in miracles, because I believe God is a supernatural God and He can do incredible things. God does use men and women who are willing and obedient according to Isaiah 1:19: *"If you are willing and obedient ye shall eat the good of the land."*

Dr. J. C. McPheeters, president of Asbury Theological Seminary, lived to be ninety-four years old. He shared that from scriptures and from his own personal experience he had learned that there are at least five miracles of healing that the Lord wants to give us: First is the miracle of instant healing. Dr. Price, an early participant in the Episcopal Healing Order of St. Luke said that in his fifty years in a ministry of healing, he had witnessed thirty-seven instant healings.

The second miracle called by Dr. McPheeters occurs when God undertakes by nature to heal us. One example is when a person cuts their thumb and it heals after cleaning it with no further interventions needed. Peter Steinke talks about the body having the capacity to heal itself—whether it is a physical body or a congregation of believers. Dr. McPheeters avowed that God undertakes to heal through doctors and nurses and medicine. He undertakes through other people to bring about a healing in our lives.

The third miracle is from God leading us to the right cure for our malady or a healing community. When it happens most of us readily confess God's guidance in this. Such was the case in the Hebrew Bible recorded in 2 Kings 20:1-11: King Hezekiah developed a boil that was spewing infection throughout his body. The prophet Isaiah told him to get his house in order because he was going to die. The king reminded God in prayer of his position in and relationship to God. God heard the prayer and sent Isaiah back to Hezekiah to give a word from the Lord that he, Hezekiah, would live and not die. Fifteen years were added to his life.

The fourth miracle occurs sometimes when we are led to a particular worship service where we hear the Word of God preached and, by a miracle of the Spirit, that word becomes God's blazing, transforming word for the day. Or sometimes it is in receiving the Holy Communion—in partaking of the bread and wine (symbolically, the body and blood of the Lord).

The fifth and last miracle Dr. Mc Pheeters discussed is the miracle of the sufficiency of God's grace. The apostle Paul had a thorn in his flesh and he wrestled with it day and night. God would not remove it. "*And lest I should be exalted above measure through the abundance of the revelations, there was given to me a thorn in the flesh, the messenger of Satan to buffer me, lest I should be exalted above measure,*" 2 Corinthians 12: 7. God did not want Paul to exalt himself through the abundance of revelations given him, so He permitted him to have the thorn in the flesh to keep him humble. According to Dake's Commentary (P. 199) this buffer was an angel of Satan, one of the spirit beings that fell with him, followed Paul and buffeted him when he was tempted to become exalted. Paul lists some things that this angel caused him to go through such as: being stoned three times, in prisons, shipwreck, in perils of the sea, surrounded by false doctrines, in hunger, thirst, and other dangerous situations.

I wish to emphasize what the prophet Isaiah was talking about when he said "willing and obedient" people would eat the good of the land. The Hebrew word for good is *toob;* its, definition includes "property, goods, goodness, fairness and beauty." It also "is used to identify the personal property of an individual . . . the plentiful harvest of the land, inward joy, the manifest goodness of the Lord . . . also a state of spiritual blessing."

The Hebrew word for land is *erets*, which "...refers to the whole earth under God's dominion. Since the earth's was God's possession, He promised to give the land of Canaan to Abraham's descendants." Israel was Abraham's descendants, and Christians are also his spiritual descendants; therefore, Isaiah 1:19 refers to those who are born again in Christ.

I have seen the Lord Jesus touch my mother over and over again in these last 12-15 years; and we always tell her she is a miracle! She says it is because we are praying for her. All of her children, grandchildren, nieces, nephews, and our friends do pray for her. She remains under the care of physicians, having been diagnosed with having severe blockage in three coronary arteries between the last 12-15 years. Dr. William Devries, the heart specialist known for putting an artificial heart, the Jarvik in at least two patients in Louisville, Kentucky, said he would not touch her for open heart surgery because she was a high risk for not making it through the surgery.

Mother was diagnosed also with a blockage in her kidney and two blockages in her legs. She traveled to Hawaii to visit my brother (a physician) and suffered two Cardiovascular Accidents or strokes while there with him; she was diagnosed with carotid arteries blocked by 90-95%. She came home . . . went to a family reunion in Atlanta and had another stroke. From these episodes she has recovered with some deficits and weakness on her side—requiring the use of a cane. She has been hospitalized numerous times but gets out and continues with her usual activities, including traveling at times with her children. She is very faithful in attending her church, and for approximately four years I was privileged to be her pastor. I encourage her to continue praising God for His love demonstrated through her to the family.

The New Testament apostles did not waste any time after they were filled with and baptized in the Holy Ghost; they immediately went around teaching, preaching, and healing. They were not afraid to operate in the gifts of the Holy Spirit because they knew the gifts were for the edification of others. God does not anoint you to twiddle your thumbs; it is so you can operate in His authority, power, and dominion. We are not to send hurt, wounded, and sick people away, but are to command them to be loosed from whatever is holding them captive. Jesus has given the Body of Christ important keys to use—the authority to bind and loose.

My first preaching message came from Mark 16:15-18 and its title was "Let's Gossip about Jesus." A friend, Elder Bill Frazier, stated that it was an unusual message to be brought forth by someone from a traditional Baptist Church, but it was the message God had given unto me. It was relatively long for an initial message—13 hand-written pages. My friend was talking about content; content for which I prayed, fasted, and sought the Lord . . . because my pastor urged me to hear from God. I agreed with Bill Frazier about the unusual content of the message—it had been over twenty years since I had heard someone talk about casting out demons. It is so important for each individual to study the Bible for their own growth and development as a Christian.

After Jesus had been resurrected, He appeared to His disciples on various occasions to encourage them and give instructions. They were in such disbelief . . . and Christ scolded them for their unbelief. Then while sitting at the table to eat with them, Jesus the Christ commissioned and instructed His disciples on how they were to go out to preach and minister:

> *And He said unto them, Go ye into all the world, and preach the gospel to every creature. He that believeth and is baptized shall be saved; but he that believeth not shall be damned. And these signs shall follow them that believe; In my name shall they cast out devils; they shall speak with new tongues; they shall take up serpents; and if they drink any deadly thing, it shall not hurt them; they shall lay hands on the sick, and they shall recover* (Mark 16:15-18).

We as born again, spirit-filled believers are to assist the person(s) in bondage and in need of deliverance; we need to discern what spirit is oppressing them and help them to understand that they can be free. For example, it may be some form of depression. Depression is a manifestation of a stronghold called *the spirit of heaviness*. We have the power to bind up the spirit of heaviness in the name of Jesus, cast it out and send it to the dry places, and loose the spirit of peace. Sometimes demons are stubborn and will try to remain because they are disembodied spirits. Use the name of Jesus and command them to come out; also plead the blood of Jesus over the person(s). I have read the Holy Word during deliverance and applied anointing oil; these things torment demons. They may speak and say this is their home but they must and will eventually come out.

How do you know when they are coming out? The person(s) will breathe them out; they may scream out, gag and cough, spit, and at times large amounts of phlegm or mucus may flow out of their mouth, absent of abdominal (stomach) contents such as food. It may start out to be small in quantity but can become large as deliverance goes forth. Sometimes I tell the altar workers to "get the bucket," to allow it to flow somewhere besides the floor. It is so awesome when God liberates someone and the person leaves your presence with the assurance that God has done this for them. How do I know? They usually verbalize it—telling what God has done before they leave our presence.

A young lady joined our church, in 1995, who had previously attended an occult church. She still had issues such as, fear, lack of trust, and other emotional problems. At that time, we had deliverance almost every time the church convened. One day while she was singing on the Praise Team, the Lord had me to look at her...and I saw a movement in her throat like a snake trying to choke her...she had begun to gag. I ran to her and commanded the spirit to come out; it obeyed, and she was free. The Kingdom of God is within us! Jesus sent His disciples out after giving instructions, saying:

> *And heal the sick that are therein and say unto them, "The Kingdom of God is come nigh (near) unto you." After they returned he said, "Behold, I give unto you*

power to tread on serpents and scorpions, and over all the power of the enemy, and nothing shall by any means hurt you" (Luke 10: 9, 19).

There are times when worship is high and as the Holy Spirit touches individuals, they may dance until they fall under the power of God. Sometimes they fall under the power of God without being touched by a person. While they are in His presence, healing does occur at times and they may rise up totally delivered. Anointed, spirit-filled worship is an avenue that is used to usher in the presence of God with power to demonstrate signs, wonders, and miracles. Miracles always point to the Lord Jesus. I believe that we are entering into a season where more miracles will be evidenced. Some people will have to see God manifest signs, wonders, and miracles before they will believe there is a true and living God—One who loves them and has given them all things pertaining to life and godliness.

In 2006 Bishop Eddie L. Long called for intercessors to meet at the Philips Arena in downtown Atlanta, for prayer. One of my colleagues shared that he asked those who needed a healing to step into the aisle. She obeyed and was immediately healed of *Meniere's disease*. Her suffering had consisted of: ringing in the ears, loss of balance, vertigo or dizziness, tinnitus (buzzing or ringing in the ears) and a sensation of fullness or pressure—all symptoms of the inner ear disturbance known as *Meniere's disease*. Dr. Henrietta (Rett) Adams informed me that she had not driven for ten years, but that day she was driving and has continued to drive. God is still performing miracles; this is just one example.

Spiritualism, 'New Age,' Buddhism, Confucianism, Hinduism, and other religions that believe in statutes, false gods, or some other doctrine founded by a mere person will not be beneficial in producing the greatest miracle—salvation of souls. When ultimately it is all said and done, you can go to heaven with a broken leg or a diseased lung, but not with a damned soul. Christ Jesus is the only way to salvation. He declared and promised, *"I am the Door; anyone who enters in through Me will be saved (will live). He will come in and he will go out [freely], and will find pasture"* (John 10:9 AMP).

We do not like to offend but the truth must be told. It will be a rude awakening to spend your whole life preparing for a better life in a new world only to find out that deception crept in to take the greatest gift from you—eternal life. When you ask Christ to be your Savior, there is a definite peace given that assures you that you no longer need to keep looking for something or someone else. This is an inner peace. Some of the turmoil on the inside of individuals comes from not having that inner peace about their salvation. Fear causes you to be tormented or restless, always looking for something to anesthetize the pain or fill the void. It is no secret what God can do; what He does for others, He will do for you.

He wants to show Himself mighty and show Himself strong on our behalf. God receives the glory whenever there is a supernatural move by Him. As you read the Acts of the Apostles and the Gospels there are so many accounts of healings that happened when Jesus arrived in the midst of hurt and broken people. "*...Jesus began to preach and to say, "Repent, for the kingdom of heaven is at hand*" (Matthew 4:17). Everyone who came to Jesus was healed. What an awesome testimony! "*Jesus Christ the same yesterday, today, and forever*" (Hebrews 13:8). Christ is always the same. "*For I am the LORD, I do not* change..." (Malachi

3:6). So that means He has not changed in His capability or desire to deliver, heal and restore us.

I submit to you that you are God's son or daughter, a rightful heir and joint heir with Christ Jesus. I believe that we as Kingdom heirs can do all things through Christ, who gives us the divine enablement to fulfill the calling that is on our life. Jesus declared to His disciples, "*Verily, verily, I say unto you, He that believeth on me, the works that I do shall he do also; and greater works than these shall he do; because I go unto my Father*" (John 14:12). He was not talking about greater miracles; rather, through Christ and the power of the Holy Spirit, the ministry of His followers would have wider spiritual effects—reaching more people than Jesus' earthly ministry did. It is already happening via high-definition technology, satellite television, the internet, radio, and through personal, as well as mass evangelism.

The following narrative reveals to us how one man needed to be forgiven so that he could be delivered from a physical ailment. He was paralyzed when he reached Jesus but left from the Lord's midst walking. Jesus came to His headquarters in Capernaum, and encountered there a man "*sick of the palsy.*" Some friends brought the man on a portable mat, to be healed. "*Jesus seeing their faith said unto the sick of the palsy; Son, be of good cheer; thy sins be forgiven thee*" (Matthew 9:2). The scribes who were present said that Jesus was blaspheming, or mocking God. The Lord was able to discern what was in their heart and He told them of their evil thoughts:

> *For whether is easier, to say, Thy sins be forgiven thee; or to say, Arise and walk? But that ye may know that the Son of man hath power on earth to forgive sins, (then saith he to the sick of the palsy,) Arise,*

> *take up thy bed, and go unto thine own house. And he arose, and departed to his house. But when the multitudes saw it, they marveled, and glorified God, which had given such power unto men* (Matthew 9:5-8).

The man did not need counseling or group therapy; he needed to be released from his sins and failures. This man needed inner (spiritual) healing for the physical healing to take place; and he was delivered and healed simultaneously.

The Dake's Bible states that "the Greek word for power is *exousia*—delegated authority and liberty to exercise the full power of attorney in all God's interests. Complete authority to act in God's stead as if God Himself were here doing the work; power to act as freely of his own will as one has power to eat and drink." Christ's power was unlimited in doing the will and works of God on earth. He now has all power in heaven and in earth, and promises to share His power with all born-again believers.

We will see signs, wonders, and miracles before the return of the Lord. Jesus did many miracles that are not recorded in the Bible. I believe certain things have not been recorded for our reading but that the Lord will do those things in our midst. It will not be anything that Jesus has not already done, but it will increase our confidence in Him and take it to another dimension. God wants to use all believers for His glory. Broken, wounded, sick, troubled, disturbed people are looking for a cure and not a 'band-aid' or temporary relief. Their desire is to be made whole, that is, delivered, healed and restored. The One who never fails a patient is the Lord Jesus. Deep inner healing is for all to receive.

NOTES

Introduction

1. Dooney da Priest, a Christian/Gospel/Rap artist of Dallas, Texas, known for the hit, "Pull Your Pants Up," www.dooneydapriest.com.
2. Holy Bible New Testament, John 14:12, King James Version.
3. Holy Bible Old Testament, Proverbs 27:17, Amplified.
4. James Strong, The New Strong's Exhaustive Concordance of the Bible (Nashville: Thomas Nelson Publishers, 2010); 2240: kairos, a Greek term meaning season or opportunity.

Chapter 1

1. Holy Bible Old Testament, Proverbs 22:6, King James Version.
2. Holy Bible New Testament, James 5:16, New Century Version.

3. Holy Bible New Testament, James 5:16, The Message Bible.
4. Holy Bible Old Testament, Proverbs 18:14, King James Version
5. Strong's Concordance, 2588: kardia, a Greek word for heart.
6. Ibid. 4937 suntribō, a Greek word for brokenhearted.
7. Finis Jennings Dake, Dake's Annotated Reference Bible King James Version, 11th ed. (Georgia: Dake Bible Sales, Inc., 1993), notes from the Targum (Book of Ruth), p. 291.
8. Trinity Broadcasting Network, film titled Ruth, www.trinitybroadcastingnetwork.
9. Holy Bible Old Testament, Ruth 1:20, 21, New International Version.
10. Dake, "Mara" means bitter, p. 291.
11. Holy Bible Old Testament, Ruth 2:2, King James Version.
12. Holy Bible Old Testament, Leviticus 19:9, 10, New International Version.
13. Holy Bible Old Testament, Ruth, Chapter 2 (paraphrased) King James Version.

Chapter 2

1. June Hunt, Counseling Through Your Bible Handbook: "Identity" (Oregon: Harvest House Publishers, 2008), p. 227.
2. Myles Monroe, Releasing Your Potential: Exposing the Hidden You, "The Tragedy of Unreleased Potential," (Shippensburg: Destiny Image Publishers, Inc., 1992), p. 25.
3. Hebrew-Greek Key Word Study Bible, King James Version, 2nd ed. (Chattanooga: AMG Publishers, 2008), 4561: sarx, a Greek term meaning flesh.

4. I Samuel 18:7, 8, King James Version.
5. Holy Bible Old Testament, Genesis 3:1-5, King James Version.
6. Holy Bible Old Testament, Genesis 3:6, King James Version.
7. Holy Bible Old Testament, Genesis 1:26-30, New Revised Standard Version.
8. Maisha Handy, "Fighting the Matrix: Toward a Womanist Pedagogy for the Black Church"; The Journal of the Interdenominational Theological Center, published, semi-annually, by the faculty of ITC in Atlanta (JITC, indexed in the ATLA Religion Database, is available in Microform through ProQuest Information and Learning Company, 2008), p. 51.
9. Donald McKim, Westminster Dictionary of Theological Terms, definition of "patriarchal" (Louisville: Westminster John Knox Press, 1996), p. 204.
10. Strong's, 3875: paraklētŏs, a Greek term for intercessor, advocate, comforter; the Holy Spirit is our Paraklētŏs. Ibid., 120: "âdâm," the Hebrew word for a human being, an individual or the species: mankind, man or person.

Chapter 3

1. Strong's Concordance, 1285 beriyth, a Hebrew word for "covenant," meaning a compact (made by passing between pieces of flesh), confederacy, covenant, league.
2. Holy Bible New Testament, Galatians 6:7, King James Version.
3. John Maxwell, The Maxwell Leadership Bible: New King James Version, "The Law of Buy-in: Moses Gains Credibility" (Nashville: Thomas Nelson, 2007), p. 84.

4. Hebrew-Greek Study Bible, 3820 labe, the Hebrew word for heart. Figuratively widely used for feelings, the will and even intellect; likewise for the emotions.
5. Michael Agnes and Charlton Laird, Webster's New World Dictionary Thesaurus, 2nd ed. (Cleveland: Wiley Publishing, Inc., 2002), p. 599. "Slave" is a human being who is owned as property by another; one dominated by some influence.
6. Holman Concise Bible Dictionary (Nashville: Broadman & Holman Publishers, 1997), p. 462. Mount Sinai means shining; called the "Mountain of God."
7. Holy Bible Old Testament, Leviticus 19:2, King James Version.
8. Hebrew-Greek Study Bible, 5303 nephilim, a Hebrew word for a feller, a bully or tyrant-giant.
9. Holy Bible Old Testament, Numbers 14:1-3, New International Version.
10. Holy Bible Old Testament, Numbers 23:19, King James Version.
11. Holy Bible New Testament, 2 Corinthians 10:5, King James Version.
12. Holy Bible New Testament, Matthew 18:18, King James Version.

Chapter 4

1. Flora Slosson Wuellner, Release: Healing From Wounds of Family, Church and Community, 2nd ed. (Nashville: Upper Room Books, 1998), p. 11.
2. Holy Bible Old Testament, Psalm 46:1, King James Version.
3. Holy Bible New Testament, 1 Corinthians 7:14, 15, King James Version.

4. Holy Bible New Testament, Luke 8:43-48, New International Version.
5. Pastoral Care, "Can Anything Good Come From this Side of the Tracks?" (Nashville: Abingdon Press), p. 44.
6. Holy Bible New Testament, Matthew 9:20-22, New International Version.
7. Holy Bible New Testament, James 2:17, New International Version.
8. Holy Bible New Testament, Romans 10:11; 16, 17, New International Version.
9. Holy Bible New Testament, Acts 10:34, Amplified.
10. Holy Bible New Testament, Matthew 27:23, 24, New International Version.
11. Dake, p. 8.
12. Ibid., 32. A Roman "scourge" is an implement used for severe punishment.
13. Holy Bible New Testament, Matthew 9:21, King James Version.
14. Strong's Concordance, 2440 himation, a Greek word for garment - Matthew 9:20.
15. Strong's Concordance, 5509 chiton, a Greek word for coat or undergarment - Matthew 5:40.
16. Strong's Concordance, 4982 sozo, a Greek word meaning whole; to save, deliver, protect (lit. or fig.) heal, preserve, save (self), do well, be (make) whole.
17. Hebrew-Greek Study Bible, 5927 aw-law, a Hebrew word meaning to mount up.
18. Holy Bible Old Testament, Isaiah 61:4, King James Version.
19. Holy Bible New Testament, Luke 10:19, King James Version.
20. Holy Bible New Testament, John 20:23, King James Version.

Chapter 5

1. Flora Slosson Wuellner discusses three major stages of healing presented in her book, Release: spiritual recovery, restoration and renewal, p. 55.
2. Holy Bible New Testament, Acts 10:38, King James Version.
3. Holy Bible New Testament, Mark 11:25-26, Amplified.
4. Holy Bible Old Testament, Proverbs 18:19, King James Version.
5. Webster's New World Dictionary and Thesaurus, "offend" Michael Agnes and Charlton Laird editors, 2nd ed. (Ohio: Wiley Publishing, Inc.), p. 442.
6. Holy Bible New Testament, 1 Peter 5:1-3, King James Version.
7. Dr. Edward P. Wimberly writes, Moving From Shame to Self-Worth, "Devastating Shame Blocks Peoples' Ability to Discern a Caring God, (Nashville: Abingdon Press, 1999), p. 71.
8. Ibid., p. 62.
9. Frances MacNutt, The Power to Heal, p. 214. "The need for inner healing usually comes forth in tears that have often been left uncried for many years."
10. Ibid., p. 214. Dr. MacNutt discusses signs and symptoms that alert the one praying that a person being prayed for needs inner healing.
11. June Hunt, p. 125.
12. Holy Bible New Testament, Ephesians 4:31, New International Version.
13. Holy Bible New Testament, 1 Peter 5:7, New International Version.
14. June Hunt, p. 126. "Even our deepest disappointments must be resolved or our bitterness will cause trouble."

15. Hunt, p. 127. Points are given on how to defeat depression (Scriptures from NIV)
    - A. "Confront any loss..." (Ecclesiastes 3:4).
    - B. "Offer your heart..." (1John 1:8-9).
    - C. "Nurture thoughts..." (Jeremiah 31:3).
    - D. "Quit negative thinking..." (Philippians 4:8).
    - E. "Understand God's Purpose ..." (Romans 8:28).
    - F. "Exchange your hurt ..." (1Thessalonians 5:18).
    - G. "Remember God is Sovereign..." (Psalm 71:5).
16. Holy Bible Old Testament, Job 2:9-10, New International Version.
17. MacNutt, p. 224. An individual discusses the freedom experienced after prayer.
18. Holy Bible New Testament, Philippians 4:6, Amplified Bible
19. Holy Bible New Testament, Romans 10:9-10, New International Version.
20. Holy Bible New Testament, Romans 10:13, New International Version.
21. Holy Bible New Testament, Matthew 6:19, Amplified.
22. Holy Bible New Testament, 1 Peter 2:24; Isaiah 53:5, New Revised Standard Version.
23. Holy Bible New Testament, I John 4:4, King James Version.
24. Holy Bible New Testament, 1 John 5:14-15, King James Version.
25. Holy Bible New Testament, Hebrews 4:12, Amplified.
26. Holy Bible Old Testament, Psalm 86:1-6, Amplified.
27. Holy Bible Old Testament, Psalm 86:7.

Chapter 6

1. Holy Bible Old Testament, Jeremiah 8: 22, Amplified.
2. Holy Bible Old Testament, Psalm 42:1-5, New Century Version.

3. Holy Bible Old Testament, Proverbs 18:14, The Message Bible.
4. Webster's Dictionary, definition for "rejection."
5. June Hunt, p. 342.
6. Ibid., p. 343.
7. Philippians 4:13, Amplified.
8. Virginia Harrison, Let it Go, (USA: Xulon Press), p. 89.
9. Ibid., p. 92.
10. Ibid., p. 94.
11. Ibid., p. 109.
12. Ibid., p. 110.
13. Ibid., p. 111.
14. Ibid., p. 112.
15. Ibid., p. 113.
16. Ibid., p. 114.
17. Ibid., p. 115.
18. Holy Bible Old Testament, Hebrews 4:15, Amplified.
19. Holy Bible Old Testament, Psalm 46:1, Amplified.
20. Holy Bible New Testament, Mark 11:24, Amplified.
21. Holy Bible New Testament, Mark 25-26, Amplified.
22. June Hunt, pp. 177-178.
23. Ibid., p. 181.
24. Flora Slosson Wuellner, p. 27.
25. Holy Bible New Testament, James 5:16, The Message Bible.
26. Holy Bible New Testament, James 4:1-2, Amplified.
27. Holy Bible New Testament, James 4:3-4, Amplified.
28. Holy Bible Old Testament, Genesis 16:1-4, Amplified.
29. Webster's New World Dictionary and Thesaurus,] definition for "contempt." p. 134.
30. Holy Bible Old Testament, Genesis 29:20-23, 25.
31. Holy Bible Old Testament, Genesis 29:25, Amplified.
32. Holy Bible Old Testament, Proverbs 6:2, Amplified.

33. Holy Bible Old Testament, Genesis 30:22-23, Amplified.
34. David A. Seamands, p. 49. "Satan's greatest psychological weapon . . . "
35. Ibid., pp. 49-54.
36. Chuck D. Pierce, The Future War of the Church, p. 257.
37. Holy Bible Old Testament, Jeremiah 9:17-20, Amplified.
38. Holy Bible Old Testament, Genesis 3:15, Amplified.
39. Chuck D. Pierce, p. 258. "Satan hates women with great wrath."
40. Holy Bible Old Testament, James 5:13, Amplified.
41. Paul Meier and Esly Regina Carvalho wrote an article for Joyce Meyers' Magazine which was also on the Internet titled, "Welcoming Inner Healing." In it they state, "... that without inner healing—the healing of the soul—people do not get to the level of holiness that God has called His church to live. www.joycemeyersministries.org.
42. Meier and Carvalho, "They often come to us in horrific emotional pain as a result of disappointments, rejections, and even personal failures—spiritual and otherwise."

Chapter 7

1. Holy Bible New Testament, Romans 14:17-19, Amplified.
2. Gwendolyn A. Washington, Faith Healing Ministry: A Christian Education Model for Clergy and Laity, (D. Min. diss., Interdenominational Theological Center, Atlanta, 2008), p.24.
3. Leonard I. Sweet, "Praying and Healing," Healing and Medicine in the Evangelical Tradition: Neither

by Might nor Power (Pennsylvania: Trinity Press International, 1994), pp. 157-158.

4. Ibid., p. 141.
5. Donald McKim, definition for term "Evangelicals," Westminster Dictionary of Theological Terms, p. 96.
6. Ibid., p. 160.
7. Holy Bible New Testament, 1 Corinthians 12:7-11, Amplified.
8. Maxie D. Dunnam, "Some Healing Is Up to You," I Am the Lord Who Heals You: Reflection On Healing, Wholeness, and Restoration (Nashville: Abingdon Press, 2004), p.16.
9. Holy Bible Old Testament, Psalm 103:1-5, King James Version.
10. Holy Bible Old Testament, Isaiah 1:19, King James Version.
11. Hebrew-Greek Bible, 2898 "toob," the Hebrew word for good.
12. Ibid., 776, erets, the Hebrew word for land.
13. Holy Bible New Testament, Mark 16:15-18, King James Version.
14. Holy Bible New Testament, Luke 10:9, 19, King James Version.
15. Holy Bible New Testament, John 10:9, Amplified.
16. Holy Bible New Testament, Matthew 4:17, King James Version.
17. Holy Bible New Testament, Hebrews 13:8, King James Version.
18. Holy Bible Old Testament, Malachi 3:6, King James Version.
19. Holy Bible New Testament, John 14: 12, King James Version.
20. Holy Bible New Testament, Matthew 9: 2, King James Version.

21. Holy Bible New Testament, Matthew 9: 5-8, King James Version.
22. Dake's Bible, commentary to Matthew 9:8, p. 8.

Faithdominion2006@yahoo.com
gwenwashingtonministries.com

CPSIA information can be obtained at www.ICGtesting.com
Printed in the USA
LVOW121606250812

295854LV00001B/2/P